THE NAKED CITY

THE NAKED CITY

True Stories and Revelations about the Real Life World
of Nursing from a Healthcare Pioneer and Author of the
Bestselling *Textbook of Basic Nursing*

Caroline Bunker Rosdahl,
RN-BC, ALA, BSN,PHN, MA

Bunker Hills Media, Minnesota USA

ISBN 9798579518057

BISAC CODES
MED058000 MEDICAL / Nursing / General
BIO017000 BIOGRAPHY & AUTOBIOGRAPHY / Medical (incl. Patients)
MED058110 MEDICAL / Nursing / Management & Leadership

BOOK COVER DESIGN by Joan Holman

Website: www.carolinerosdahl.com

Bunker Hills Media
PO Box 41307
Minneapolis, Minnesota 55441-0307

CONTENTS

PREFACE

You ought to write a book," my good friend and nursing colleague said.

I laughed, "Ha, ha! As you know, I already wrote a book. I've updated it ten times in the past fifty years since I first wrote it. It's now well over 2,000 pages. So I don't feel a need to write any more books."

She said, "I know, I know. Your *Textbook of Basic Nursing* is a classic in the nursing profession and your name is legendary. But I think you should write another kind of a book. A record of your life as a nurse."

I sighed, "Sounds like a lot of work to me. And I'm not sure anyone would want to read it."

"I think lots of people would want to read it. You've had an amazing career in the nursing profession, spanning many decades. From the mid twentieth century through present day nursing in the twenty-first century. You didn't retire but continued to work in the field. You have witnessed so many changes throughout the years and have a lot of insights about the nursing profession."

My friend continued, "You have worked with some of the top surgeons and history makers in the field of medicine. I think many people would really enjoy your book.

"Especially those interested in going into the nursing profession, as well as those already in the nursing or medical field.

"And your life shows how one's career path might take unexpected and wonderful twists and turns.

"And your true stories give a glimpse into the often strange and unusual expressions of the human experience that nurses can encounter in their work."

Okay, so I have now written the book:

***The Naked City: True Stories and Revelations about the Real Life World of Nursing from A Healthcare Pioneer and Author of the Bestselling* Textbook of Basic Nursing**

This book is much shorter than my textbook.

And I've written it in such a way that you can read it in bits and pieces.

It's full of lots of stories and anecdotes.

And it includes many historical photos.

Thankfully, I have been blessed to be able to make a positive and far-reaching contribution.

I sincerely hope my new book can benefit you in some way, whether as education, inspiration, or even entertainment.

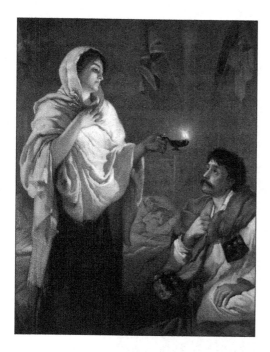

The Lady with the Lamp—
Honored as the Founder of
Modern Nursing and an icon
of Victorian culture, Florence
Nightingale gave nursing
a favorable reputation and
became known as "The Lady
with the Lamp," because she
made rounds with wounded
soldiers at night during the
Crimean War. (1891 painting
by Henrietta Rae)

NIGHTINGALE PLEDGE

(1935 revised version—Wikipedia)

- I solemnly pledge myself before God and in the presence of this assembly to pass my life in purity and to practice my profession faithfully.

- I will abstain from whatever is deleterious and mischievous, and will not take or knowingly administer any harmful drug.

- I will do all in my power to maintain and elevate the standard of my profession and will hold in confidence all personal matters committed to my keeping and all family affairs coming to my knowledge in the practice of my calling.

- With loyalty will I aid the physician in his work, and as a missioner of health, I will dedicate myself to devoted service for human welfare."

The Nightingale Pledge is included in ceremonies for all nurses graduating from a nursing program. "United States nurses have recited the pledge at pinning ceremonies for decades. In recent years, many US nursing schools have made changes to the original or 1935 versions." (Wikipedia)

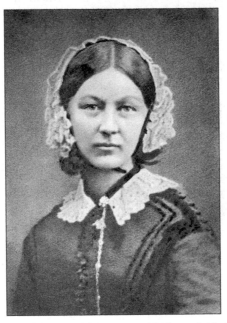

Florence Nightingale (May 12, 1820–August 13, 1910)

"When she was twenty-four, Florence indicated her interest in the nursing profession, but her parents were strongly opposed. It needs to be noted that, in the nineteenth century, nurses did not enjoy the reputation that they enjoy today. In fact, the reputation they enjoy today is largely due to the reforms brought about by Florence Nightingale."

(From Hamilton, *Florence Nightingale, A Life Inspired*)

FOREWORD

This year of 2020 marks the premier publication of the distinguished nursing profession pioneer Caroline Bunker Rosdahl's new book, *The Naked City: True Stories and Life Experiences of a Healthcare Pioneer and Bestselling Author of the Landmark Textbook of Basic Nursing*. Coincidentally, the year of 2020 has been designated as the *International Year of the Nurse and Midwife* by the World Health Organization in honor of the 200th anniversary of the birth of Florence Nightingale, renowned as the *Founder of Modern Nursing*.

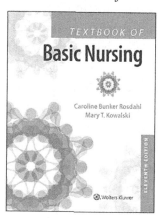

Textbook of Basic Nursing, Edition 11 (50th Anniversary)

And also, coincidentally, the year 2020 is the year of the Covid-19 pandemic, which has put into the limelight the heroic efforts of many dedicated nurses who serve on the front lines of what can be a dangerous profession.

This collection of Rosdahl's true life experiences, shared through her stories and commentary, gives an interesting historical look at what it has been like to be a nurse in America in a time period spanning more than a half century, from post WWII to the modern era.

The year 2020 also marks the fifty-three year anniversary of the publication of Rosdahl's perennial international classic *Textbook of Basic Nursing*, now in its eleventh edition.

A Look Inside the "Naked City" of Nursing

An acclaimed healthcare leader, practicing nurse, educator, administrator, innovator, and major contributor to the nursing profession, Rosdahl has had decades of an insider's look at human life in its rawest form.

As she can tell you, being a nurse presents many different types of experiences and can give you not just a glimpse, but a full frontal look behind the curtain, where the human experience is exposed and which includes the good, the bad, the ugly, the wild and unbelievable and often the very strange and bizarre.

During her long career and in her various roles as a hospital nurse, a public health nurse, an educator, a school nurse visiting rural one-room schoolhouses (in the "olden" days), and being a nurse in a mental health unit, Rosdahl has seen it all.

Rosdahl worked with such legendary top surgeons as Dr. C. Walton Lillehei, world-renowned as the "Father of Open-Heart Surgery," and Dr. Owen Wangensteen, who developed the Wangensteen tube, which used suction to treat small bowel obstruction, an innovation estimated to have saved a million lives by the time of his death in 1981.

Under Dr. Wangensteen's leadership, University of Minnesota surgeons, including Dr. Lillehei, played leading roles in pioneering open-heart surgery. Dr. Wangensteen was Chief of Surgery at the University of Minnesota for thirty-seven years, and medical students from all over the world were attracted to the department because of his strong emphasis on research and laboratory experiments.

From witnessing medical history being made at the University of Minnesota hospital, to being on the scene in her off hours where she was involved in rescuing and/or attending to victims of serious automobile accidents or medical emergencies, to interacting with high profile murderers in a mental health unit where she worked as a nurse, Rosdahl has had a lifetime of service, both on-duty and off-duty.

As Rosdahl says, "Once a nurse, always a nurse."

The Nursing Profession

During the time period since Rosdahl first started working as a nurse, the field of nursing has grown and evolved and gone through tremendous change. One thing that has not changed is that although many more men have become nurses, it is still a profession that is predominantly female.

- In 1937, the year Rosdahl was born, there were approximately 300,000 "professional" nurses in the United States, of which ninety six percent were women. (*Journal of Clinical Nursing: Counting Nurses, The Power of Historical Census Data*)

- Today, in 2020, there are over four million Registered Nurses in the United States. And although there has been an increase in the percentage of male nurses, over ninety two percent of nurses are still women. (*American Nurses Association*)

- Nursing continues to be popular and today being a Registered Nurse is the #2 leading occupation of employed women. (*United States Department of Labor*)

When Rosdahl was born May 15, 1937 in Sauk Centre, Minnesota, the world was a very different place.
Especially for women.

- Only eleven percent of women worked in 1930. (*US Census*)

- Only 25.4 percent of women over the age of fourteen worked in 1940. Three quarters of these women worked as schoolteachers or nurses. (*US Census*)

- The United States entered WWII on December 7, 1941, and by the mid-1940s, the percentage of women in the American work force had expanded from twenty five percent to thirty six percent.

- Only seventeen years before Rosdahl was born, women in the United States got the national legal right to vote when the

Nineteenth Amendment became part of the U.S. Constitution on August 18, 1920.

A Half-Century of Dramatic Change

During her lifetime since the 1930s, Rosdahl has witnessed dramatic changes in her profession and in the way Americans live and work. Innovations in technology not only changed the world of medicine, but also transformed American life through the fields of transportation, communications and other areas.

In the past sixty-plus years, the working climate for women has also experienced dramatic changes.

Today most women work outside the home, and women have experienced progress in earnings and in education as well as in having greater opportunities in managerial and professional occupations.

Pay equity for women has increased, although it still is not on par with men's salaries.

- It was reported in 2014 that nearly six in ten women aged sixteen and older (fifty seven percent) worked outside the home. (*U.S. Bureau of Labor Statistics*)

- In 1937, women's average annual pay was $525, just over half the average annual pay of $1,027 for men. (*Social Security Administration*)

- Today, women in the United States earn a median annual income of approximately $45,097 annually, which is eighty one percent of men's median annual income of $55,291. (*Catalyst. org. Statistics for 2018*)

- Today, the average annual salary for a Registered Nurse in the United States is $73,550.

- Today, being a Registered Nurse is the #2 leading occupation of employed women. (*United States Department of Labor*)

Lightening the Load Through Humor and Storytelling

Nurses have stressful jobs. Frequently overworked and overburdened, they must still provide the nurturing and strength to help others through their caregiving and service. Compassion and meaningful connection with patients can be an antidote to the problems encountered in the profession. And humor, storytelling, and laughter can also be great antidotes, helping to lighten the load and uplift the spirit.

Rosdahl's great sense of humor is shared through many of the stories in her book.

Rosdahl's Major Industry Changing Innovation

Over a half century ago, Rosdahl introduced something unique, something never used in nursing education before. She introduced the use of behavioral objectives into her development of a Practical Nursing Program at a technical school in the largest school district in Minnesota.

After implementing the program, the Minnesota Board of Nursing began recommending her course materials to other schools and the materials eventually became used throughout Minnesota and worldwide. Behavioral objectives are now written for all nursing programs at all levels. These objectives were a key reason Rosdahl was asked to write her major nursing textbook.

So Rosdahl forever changed the field of nursing education. The use of the behavioral objectives she introduced into widespread nursing education over fifty years ago continues in present day nursing. These objectives were incorporated into her classic basic nursing textbook and in addition to approval by the Minnesota Board of Nursing, her program received national accreditation by the National League for Nursing (NLN).

From the Past to the Present

Rosdahl's respected and popular educational textbook and ancillary educational tools have incorporated the changes in the nursing profession and made them relevant for the modern nurse. When Rosdahl first started her professional career, many nurses were trained through extensive clinical experience. They received on-the-job training in hospital diploma schools. Most students took care of patients and learned on the job. Nursing students sometimes worked long shifts in hospitals, often with minimal clinical supervision.

She says, *"Today so much of the education is in the laboratory with simulation. There are actually programs without any hands-on clinical experience, and that to me, is really scary because the students graduate without any idea of how to relate to a patient."*

Today, graduates enter the workforce and experience a "culture shock," where they are not used to working weekends, long shift hours, and interacting with patients.

An Interesting Footnote

The year 2020 also marks the 100-year anniversary of the first publication of the acclaimed American classic book *Main Street* by Sinclair Lewis, one of America's most important twentieth century authors.

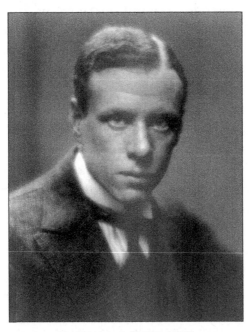

Sinclair Lewis (1885-1951)

Lewis was the first American author to be awarded the Nobel Prize for distinction in world literature.

It turns out that Caroline Rosdahl and Sinclair Lewis share some interesting things in common.

- Both authors share the same birthplace and childhood home of Sauk Centre, Minnesota.

- Both authors wrote perennially popular books spanning decades and which have been read by countless numbers of individuals throughout the world.

- In a world where very few authors are ever successful, by any measure of success, Caroline Bunker Rosdahl and Sinclair Lewis are extraordinarily successful authors.

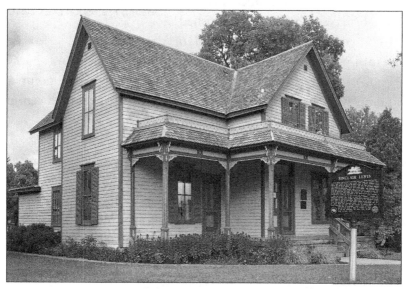

Boyhood Home of Sinclair Lewis, Sauk Centre, Minnesota

Main Street: The Story of Carol Kennicott, a novel that satirized small town life and which drew upon his roots growing up in Sauk Centre, is perhaps Sinclair Lewis's most famous book, and the book that led in part to his eventual 1930 Nobel Prize for Literature.

The novel instantly made Lewis a wealthy man and an international sensation. It sold 180,000 copies in just over six months, and it is estimated that two million Americans read it before his next book was published in 1922.

Lewis's hometown of Sauk Centre served as the inspiration for Gopher Prairie, the fictional setting for his enormously popular *Main Street*, the first of his great literary successes that established him as an important figure in twentieth century American literature and the most famous American novelist of the 1920s.

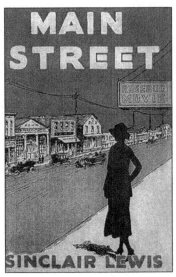

Main Street Book Dust Cover, First Edition, 1920

Main Street was an immediate, phenomenal success when it was published. By 1921, you could see a copy of *Main Street* in almost any parlor of any boarding house in the country. It was the book of the century and the best-selling novel up to that point and the number one bestseller for the first quarter of the twentieth century. And it continued to sell at a steady pace for decades after that.

The name of the strong female central character in *Main Street* is Carol (Milford) Kennicott, a bright, college-educated woman with progressive ideas. Not unlike Caroline Bunker Rosdahl.

Most certainly, baby Caroline Bunker was born into a family that was familiar with Sinclair Lewis since his book published in 1920 had put Sauk Centre on the map, so to speak, and Caroline's father Frank Bunker, a published poet, and Sinclair Lewis' father Edwin (E.J.), were good friends.

As early as the 1925-26 school year, because of the book's popularity, high school teams from Sinclair Lewis's hometown of Sauk Centre began to be called the *Main Streeters*. The Sauk Centre High School still goes by that name.

Lewis moved away from Sauk Centre at the age of seventeen in 1902 to attend a college preparatory school on the East Coast. He eventually graduated from Yale University in 1908, and only returned to his hometown for visits. When he died in 1951, his cremated ashes were buried in Sauk Centre. And Rosdahl attended Lewis's funeral.

The small central Minnesota town of Sauk Centre has paid homage to Sinclair Lewis and established a historic house museum and National Historic Landmark of his boyhood home.

The Sinclair Lewis Foundation acquired Lewis's boyhood house in 1956 and restored it to how it looked during his boyhood. They offer tours regularly during the summer and by appointment throughout the rest of the year.

The original 3rd Street in Sauk Centre has been renamed "Sinclair Lewis Avenue" and Main Street is now named "The Original Main Street." When *Main Street* came out in 1920, the population of Sauk Centre was just over 3,000, which is still what it is today.

So it turns out that Caroline Bunker Rosdahl shares the stage with a successful historic fellow American author and will go down as an important historical figure, not only in her native town, and native state, but also throughout the world.

Her classic textbook has sold countless copies over the past fifty-three years since it was first published, and continues to be re-printed and sold worldwide. It would be a conservative estimate to say that her seminal book has impacted millions of lives in the nursing profession and those that they serve.

In a world where very few books ever published sell more than a few thousand copies in their lifetime, *Textbook of Basic Nursing* and *Main Street* stand out as two of the bestselling books in history.

And Sauk Centre natives Caroline Rosdahl and Sinclair Lewis have earned historical status as two of the bestselling authors in the world in the past 100 years.

When asked about the future of nursing, Rosdahl says she sees a very bright future that however will grow more complicated over time and have a need for more specialized nurses and more nurses in the community.

Might I add that as people are sent home early from hospitals and with an aging population, they will need to be cared for from a home environment. Consequently, I would highly recommend that every home have a copy of Rosdahl's *Textbook of Basic Nursing*.

When I first received the book I was really excited about it and told my husband that it would be an excellent reference book for every family and in every home. It provides a comprehensive education that could be helpful in any number of situations.

As we move towards self-care, it has never been more important to engage in self-education about our bodies and well being.

The Naked City is a valuable historical overview of the field of nursing from a landmark figure in the profession, presented in an entertaining and interesting format with many true-life stories from her decades working in the field of nursing.

Caroline's formidable spirit of service and commitment to excellence as well as her great personality and sense of humor, shine through the pages of the book.

Joan Holman, M.A.

- Author, Producer, Acclaimed Internet Guru

- Author of *Hands That Touch, Hands That Heal,* the biography of renowned massage pioneer Sister Rosalind Gefre (Sister Rosalind Christian Ministries 2003)

- Featured notable woman in the book *Dear Success Seeker: Wisdom from Outstanding Women* (Simon & Schuster 2009)

- Creator of the PBS Television Program *The Legacy of Achievement* (Featuring the Lives and Legacies of Great Achievers)

INTRODUCTION
A MESSAGE FROM THE AUTHOR

RHEUMATIC FEVER: When I was four-years-old, I had rheumatic fever. I spent nearly a year in bed and even had a short stay at Children's Hospital in St. Paul. (There were glass dividers between the beds in the ward. The little girl in the cubicle next to me died and everyone tried to hide the fact, but we knew.)

I turned five while I was still on bed-rest. Can you imagine trying to keep a small child in bed?

My parents and caregivers read to me and played with me and I learned to read when I was very young. Because of everyone's diligence, I have had no negative after-effects, for which I am very grateful.

MY ROLE MODEL: Our pastor's wife was a Registered Nurse (Mrs. Runion) and she came some days to help take care of me. She showed up in her starched white uniform, Cuban-heeled white shoes, white nylons with the back seam, and her perky nurses' cap. She became my idol and I wanted to be a nurse for the rest of my childhood. It was a fortunate decision because in those days, girls were usually secretaries, teachers, or diploma nurses. I wanted to go to college. When I graduated from high school, I went on to fulfill my dream of becoming a nurse. (And, I also made it into the University Band!)

THE QUARANTINE: In addition to rheumatic fever, I had all the childhood diseases, including measles. I remember being quarantined in my home. (There were no preventive vaccinations for measles at that time.)

During the quarantine, there was a big red sign on our door that said, **Quarantine! Do Not Enter.**

My father had to stay with the Andersens next door, or he would not have been allowed to work. I remember waving to him out the window as he went to and from work.

MY FATHER: My father and I span nearly 140 years. He remembered the first car that came to Sauk Centre and the first flight of the Wright Brothers in December, 1903. (He was nineteen years old at the time.) I have observed hyperbaric medicine, jet planes, open-heart surgery, the Space Shuttle, and the first person to walk on the moon. And, I also have observed many other amazing advances in medicine and surgery.

All the incidents in this book are totally true.

And, all but a very few *actually happened to me* (or were witnessed by me.)

My career has spanned many years and has touched several very different settings. One of my goals in writing this book relates to the future.

I want nurses to realize the myriad of options and adventures open to them.

A nursing career has multiple facets; there is absolutely no need ever to become bored. And, nursing occurs everywhere, not just in a clinic or hospital.

Illness is not funny. It is serious business. People are often frightened or confused.

Sometimes, people don't make it. However, some things patients and families (and staff) do or say are humorous. Some incidents are very sad. I do not in any way intend to demean or insult anyone with these stories. But, sometimes these stories help us to gain insight into human nature. And, sometimes we need to add a little humor, in order to survive a difficult or frightening situation. There are so many stories from my nursing career, I could not begin to tell them all.

The title of this book comes from a *true story* in my experience.

The Psych Patient Who Thought He Could Fly

Late one *very cold winter night*, a male psych patient demanded to leave. Since he was on a hold, he could not legally be discharged from the hospital. I explained this to him and in the next minute, I saw him running down the length of the third floor-nursing unit, with me running right behind him. He smashed through the window of the patient ward at a dead run and never missed a beat, as he landed in a bush and a snowbank, and took off running down 7th Street in Minneapolis.

I called the police and they asked, "Is there any way we could recognize him?"

I said "Well, he is probably the only man running down the street in an open-backed hospital gown and paper slippers!" It didn't take long for the police to locate him and bring him back to the hospital.

This incident gave me the idea for *The Naked City*. I have had many adventures in the Naked City. This book offers a sampling.

I couldn't possibly make up this stuff!

PLEASE NOTE: In a few cases, I have changed names to protect the privacy of patients/clients and staff.

AUTHOR DISCLAIMER: It is important to remember that Sinclair Lewis was writing in the early 1900s. His beliefs and prejudices reflect much of the thinking of the times. His comments about "Swedes" and "Germans" and "Negroes" and "women" indicate lifestyles and mores of the time. The author of *The Naked City does not* hold these prejudices and does not agree with Lewis' characterization of the people that he knew. Please keep this in mind when reading books by Lewis.

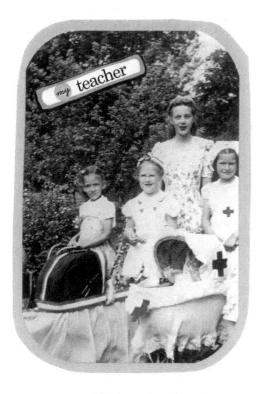

Three childhood friends and future nurses with Miss Hammerstein, their teacher, in 1943—Caroline, Jane, and Dona (BH Media)

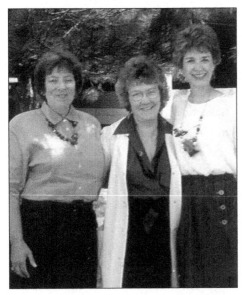

Three childhood friends who are graduate RNs FiftyYears Later—Caroline, Jane, and Dona (BH Media)

DEDICATION

This book is dedicated to all the nurses and health care workers who risk their lives to care for others.

To all the educators who have taught these nurses, including Katherine Densford Dreeves, Director of the University of Minnesota School of Nursing from 1930 to 1959. It was her vision and leadership that guided us into a rewarding and lifelong nursing career. She was a visionary; her work led to the building of a school that was and is a leader in nursing education.

And to Connie White Delaney, the current Professor and Dean of the School of Nursing. She and her staff have advanced nursing education to a totally new level. The school is now recognized as one of the premier nursing schools in the country.

And to all the nurses who have come before and who will follow.

"We, as faculty, have been forced to develop new teaching/learning strategies . . . learning is transferable to many settings, including virtual learning."—C. Delaney, Town Hall Meeting, University of Minnesota, 5-20-2020.

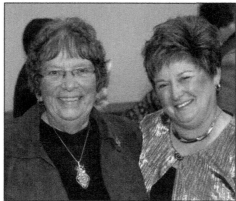

Caroline Rosdahl and Professor/Dean Connie White Delaney, 2009
(Keith Bunker Rosdahl)

ACKNOWLEDGMENTS

I wish to express my sincere thanks to those who have supported my personal and professional development.

My father, Frank Bunker, was a poet; my mother was a teacher. They encouraged me to follow in their footsteps. One cannot omit my husband, Ron Christensen, and our children and grandchildren; Keith, Kim, Bailey, and Emily; Kathy, Jeff, Sam, Allie, Megan, Mary, and Erin; Gary, Kizzy, Matthew, Abbi, and Jesse (and the great-grand-children); and Mark (1950-2019: R.I.P.) Thanks!

My dear friend, Betty Paul Sporleder (1937-2018), an English and speech teacher, always believed in me and encouraged me. She is proofreading for me in Heaven. Rest well GGB.

Joan Holman, a book consultant and mentor. She has guided me through the entire process of self-publishing. She has listened to my whining and frustration. She praised my successes. And, she has referred me to other people who could help. Nothing would have happened without Joan.

Jon-Mikel VanDerWege, my computer consultant. I could never have waded through the technology without him.

Special thanks to Judy Johnson Miller, RN, BSN, MA, for reviewing the manuscript. A distinguished nursing profession

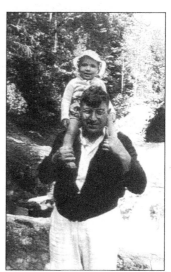

"Daddy" and Caroline, 1938
(BH Media)

leader, Judy served as Director of the Maternal-Child Health Division for the Visiting Nurse Association (VNA) of Central New Jersey, and later as the Quality Improvement Specialist for the state of New Jersey.

Illona Iris, the beta reader. Her suggestions were invaluable. And she helped process the photos.

Mary Gartamaker, who relieved me of housekeeping tasks, so I could devote my time to writing.

And, last but not least, my beloved pets. My first kitty was Scampy Fluffy Bunker; she has been followed by many other cats and dogs. My first dog, Zipper, was my constant companion during my lonely early childhood. Also, two of my sweet kitties, (Little Orphan) "Annie," and her stepmother, Miss Kitty (aka "Futtzie.") They were both rescue cats and brought us many years of love. Annie went from six ounces to six pounds (after the Vet said she would not live,) but we nursed her along and she

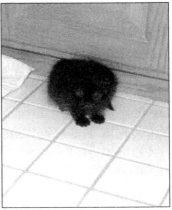

"Baby Annie": Six ounces—these are four-inch tiles

lived for nineteen and a half years! I believe my nursing experience helped save her. Now, we have a mom "Patches," and her ten-month-old kitten, "Goldie" (aka "Punkin.") They were found in the woods, abandoned, *with ten kittens in twenty below zero weather.*

And, to all the patients, who allowed me to share in their health care.

There are millions of stories in the NAKED CITY. A few of them are presented here. And the beat goes on.

Nursing is everywhere. Once a nurse, always a nurse.

CHAPTER 1

NURSING ASSISTANT

St. Michael's Hospital

I decided to become a professional nurse at age four. So, becoming a nursing assistant was a logical first step.

St. Michael's Hospital in Sauk Centre, Minnesota, was a small fifty-bed Catholic Hospital. It was run by the nuns and (I later learned) only employed Catholic nurses and other staff, even though it was sponsored by the city. (I was Protestant.)

I applied to work there as a nurse's aide/nursing assistant and was not hired, even though some of my friends were. I did not understand. I needed to make money, so I did baby-sitting for twenty-five cents an hour in the early 1950s. Then, I worked at Grossman's Variety Store for thirty-five cents an hour. (Mr. Grossman trusted me—a fifteen-year-old—and left me to run the store while he went on vacation.)

Occasionally, I also helped my Aunt Pearle run the Cream Station in LaPorte, Minnesota.

This was a subsidiary of the Bemidji Creamery.

Local dairy farmers would bring in their large cans of milk. These weighed about 100 pounds; (and so did I!) I can't believe I lifted those heavy cans. We tested the milk for butter fat content and the farmers were paid based on the percentage of butter fat in their milk. This was a great introduction for me to laboratory testing and also to relationships with the farmers.

My Introduction to St. Michael's

My father had a heart attack when I was a sophomore in high school. I was pulled out of gym class by the principal, Mr. Thompson, who immediately drove me to the hospital in my gym clothes.

A nun met me at the door and informed me that I would not be admitted to see my father "until I put on more appropriate clothing," (even though I didn't know how my Dad was doing.)

So, I had to go back to the school and change out of my gym shorts into regular street clothes.

I was very frightened, upset, and angry, but I guess I was polite. (I still can't believe they couldn't find a gown or something for me to wear.)

The Protestant Test Case

Not long after this, the city fathers complained to the hospital about only hiring Catholic girls to be nurses' aides/assistants. (I did not know this until years later.) It was supposed to be a *community hospital.*

So, one day I received a call asking if I still wanted to work at the hospital. I jumped at the chance and was very excited. I worked every weekend and some days after school. I worked full time during the summer and during school vacations, often being assigned to split shifts, so my entire day was taken up with the hospital. Here, I got forty *cents an hour!* And I loved it.

Years later, I was talking to Sister Martha, one of the nuns, and she told me how I came to be hired. She remembered the incident with my father (and was, no doubt, the nun who had met me at the door.) She had been impressed by how I handled the situation, even though she knew I was very upset, angry, and frightened. She had recommended me to be hired as the first Protestant nurses' aide. So, I was the "*Protestant test case.*" I had no idea everyone was watching to see how I would do. And I was not aware I was the test case until years later.

The hospital made sure I went to my own church every Sunday. They did not want any repercussions. I was required to leave at 10:30 AM and could not come back until 12:30 PM. (Our church was at 11:00.) They didn't know if I went to church or not, but they made sure I was available, so no one could complain.

A retired priest, Father Gauthier, was the resident Chaplain of the hospital. One day he said to me, "You're the little Protestant girl, aren't you?"

When I said I was, he said, "Well, you can pray anyway!"

On-The-Job "Training"

I had *absolutely no orientation* to the job at the hospital. They knew I wanted to be a nurse, so I guess they assumed I knew what to do, by "osmosis." My very first day, *immediately after I walked in*, I was sent in to clean the delivery room after a delivery. They gave me no instructions. If that didn't scare me away, nothing would!

They had me do everything while I was a nurses' aide/assistant. I passed oral medications. I don't remember giving shots, but I monitored the progress of IVs. Sometimes, I was the only staff member on a nursing unit.

I remember doing special duty for several days with a huge man who was having DTs (delirium tremens) while detoxifying from alcohol. Some of his friends came and helped me *hold him down*. (There was *no medication protocol* in those days.) I now know that this can be a very life-threatening situation, but I didn't know it then. Fortunately, the patient made it through.

Rules and Procedures

The nuns were very concerned about appearances. For example, the window shades had to be pulled down exactly the same distance, so their bottoms were even and level. The bedspread had to be exactly parallel with the floor. Great emphasis was placed on appearances.

STORIES

I clearly remember many of my experiences as a Nursing Assistant. Following are some examples.

The Tangled Bike

Sister Martha was quite young. One day, she borrowed someone's bicycle. (All the nuns wore full-length habits, with veils and coifs covering their heads.) While she was riding the bike, Sister Martha's habit got caught in the chain. She had to walk back to the hospital, carrying the bike.

She specifically asked me to help untangle her. I later realized that this was probably because I was the only non-Catholic staff person. She was very embarrassed and made me promise not to tell Mother Superior. (She may have gotten in trouble for talking to me, a secular.)

Retrieving the Body

There was a terrible boating accident on Sauk Lake and a gentleman drowned. I was assigned to go with the ambulance to pick up the body after it was recovered by divers. That was a very sad event that a sixteen-year-old nursing assistant will never forget!

The Terrible Burn Case

In those days, many auto service garages did not have hoists. They used a pit in the ground. When the mechanics wanted to fix the bottom of a car, they drove the car over the pit and then climbed down into the pit.

One day, a mechanic in town decided to clean out the pit with a blowtorch. Unfortunately, the pit was full of oil, gas fumes, and other debris. When he lit the torch, the whole thing exploded. This was the worst burn I have ever seen in my entire life, including during the rest of my nursing career.

The man was transferred to a hospital in the Twin Cities and he lived; however, it was a miracle.

Sister Agnes

The Anesthetist at St. Michael's was Sister Agnes. She was very dignified and formal. She ran a very disciplined Operating Room (OR.) Since Sister Agnes was the only anesthetist in the hospital, she felt very important. Dr. Julian DuBois (aka "Dr. Judy") called her "Aggie" and she absolutely hated that, but she couldn't do anything about it, because he was a doctor and she was "only a nurse."

Peter Rabbit

I had a small stuffed animal I dearly loved. My mother thought I was too old for it and would take him away from me and put him away. He had become very worn and ragged. My mother had also made him a pair of pants, because his pants were frayed. (We can't have a naked rabbit, you know!)

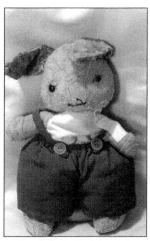

Peter Rabbit was Caroline's constant companion when she had rheumatic fever (CB Rosdahl)

Then, I would get sick and Dr. Judy would come to our house. He would always ask where Peter Rabbit was and then my mother would have to dig him out and give him back to me. And, then she would have to begin the process of taking him away again. (I don't know why she didn't just let me keep him.) And, I'm sure Dr. Judy did this just to irritate my mother. (I still have Peter Rabbit.)

What Would People Think?

My mother spent a lot of her life worrying about "What would the neighbors think?" One day a local gentleman named Charlie, who everyone knew had a problem with alcohol, passed out on our lawn.

My mother made my father drag Charlie next door, so nobody would think he was our friend or related to us. I can't imagine what the neighbor thought. (Maybe, Charlie was dragged further up the block?)

Being an "O.W."

In those days, having a baby without being married was a big deal and was often considered a disgrace to the family. People often "had to get married" if they were pregnant (or were forced to give up the baby for adoption.) Some of these "shot-gun" marriages survived, but many didn't.

If a single pregnant woman came into the hospital, she was classified as an "O.W." (*out of wedlock.*) OW was written in large letters on her chart and in the Kardex (the card file containing nursing instructions for each patient.) There were also "homes for unwed mothers," one of which was In the Twin Cities. It was called "Booth Memorial Hospital" and was run by the Salvation Army.

Many people today choose to have children without being married. It allows single women to be mothers without requiring that they "find a man." In addition, many couples choose to live together and perhaps have children, without being married. It is important for the nurse to remain unbiased and to accept all peoples' life styles.

The High School Inconsistency

One of my high school classmates became pregnant during our senior year. She and her boy friend went together to the Principal and told him they wanted to get married. She was told she would not be allowed to stay in school *if she got married*, although her boy friend could stay. So, she remained single, finished the school year, and was hugely pregnant at graduation.

Another girl wanted to get married before her boy friend was sent overseas in the Army. She was not allowed to continue in school in Sauk Centre, because she was married. So she drove twenty-five miles one-way to a neighboring high school (Glenwood) and was able to graduate.

I personally was disturbed by these unfair practices. Today, high schools have programs and child care for young mothers. In addition, young women are allowed to be married and complete their education.

The Secret

One day, a girl from another town came home to spend a weekend with her parents. She worked in the "Cities" (Minneapolis/St. Paul) and was several years out of high school. I did not know her. The girl was tall, thin, and *single*.

She began having severe stomach cramps and her parents thought she was having an appendicitis attack. When she got to the hospital, it was discovered that she was in labor; she delivered a full-term baby. (She did *not* look pregnant.)

The nuns took me into a room, backed me up to the wall, and warned me that "*God would strike me dead if I ever told anyone!*" The child was raised by his grandmother. I have no idea if anyone ever found out about it.

The Beginning of My Nursing Education

I loved my work at the hospital and it served to solidify my desire to be a nurse. I also returned home after my freshman year in college and worked full time at the hospital. I did get a lot of valuable experience, although it was a "self-study program." I do think I pretty much learned to do things right and didn't have to "unlearn" things during my nursing program.

Several of my best friends also became nurses (Dona, Jeannie, Jane, and Geri.) They all went to three-year hospital-based nursing programs and had to return to college for advanced degrees. I wanted to go to the University of Minnesota, partly *because I wanted to be in the band.* In addition, I wanted to go to a Big Ten school (and football games, etc.)

I was part way through my *five-year nursing program* before I realized I would get a college degree, in addition to the RN, and my friends wouldn't. (At the University, we had two years of college—basic courses—and then a three-year "training program" on top of that.)

Going to the U. was a very *fortunate accident*, because the Bachelor's degree has helped me immensely throughout my career. (Most nurses in those days did not get a college degree and there were no two-year programs yet.) The program at the University, guided by Katherine Densford, was excellent.

And, I also was able to be in the band. (Chapters 2 and 6)

I am still associated with the University of Minnesota Band as a Director on the Alumni Band Board. And, my son was in the Band when he was in college at the U. In the fall seasons of 2018 and 2019, my twin granddaughters were also in the Marching Band at the U. So, we *had three generations on the field at the Homecoming halftime,* with the current band and the Alumni Band. This had never occurred before.

The Army Connection

I wanted to join the Army after high school and become an Army Nurse. However, everyone I knew, including my boyfriend and my family said, "Absolutely not!" (At that time, some people frowned on having women in the Armed Forces.)

It was very sad, because my education would have been paid for and I would have been a Lieutenant upon graduation. So, I did not join the Army and I worked my way through college.

Later, I met a very important Army Nurse, Clara Adams-Ender, who was a few years younger than I. She was born in North Carolina, one of ten children in a sharecropper's family, living on a tobacco farm. Her father encouraged her to join the Army so she could become a

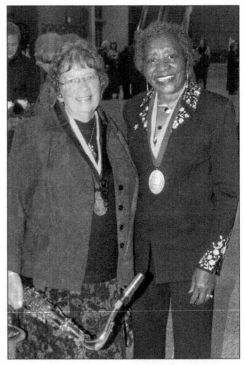

Caroline Rosdahl and Brigadier General Clara Adams-Ender wearing the Centennial medals received, 2009 (Keith Bunker Rosdahl)

8

nurse, because her family could not afford to send her to college. She received her Bachelor's Degree at a local Carolina college and later a Master's Degree in Nursing at the University of Minnesota.

Adams-Ender held a number of important positions. She rose through the Army ranks, working at Walter Reed Army Medical Center and teaching nursing. She was the first woman to receive a Master of Military Art and Science Degree at the U.S. Army Command College in Kansas. She also graduated from the U.S. Army War College, the first African American nurse to do so. She held many very important positions and became a Brigadier General. She was *Chief of the United States Army Nurse Corps* from 1987 to 1991 and was later the Commanding General of Fort Belvoir in Virginia.

Adams-Ender received many honors and awards, including being named one of the 350 women "who changed the world" by *Working Women* magazine. She was Grand Marshal of the Minnesota Homecoming Parade and, along with me, was also named as one of the *100 Distinguished Alumni of the University of Minnesota* at the Centennial Celebration in 2009. (Chapter 2)

The Reason for Being a Nurse

Throughout my career, I have met many memorable people. I certainly feel I have helped some of them. But most often, you never know. Occasionally however, a former patient provides thanks and gives you an additional reason to continue being a nurse. Following is an example. (See also Chapter 12)

CRY
Sometimes when I am alone, I cry because I am on my own.
The tears I cry are bitter and warm. They flow with life, but
take no form.
I find it difficult just to carry on, so I can find out where I
belong.
If I had a tear that I could send, it would be to my treasured
friend.

The world moves fast, it would rather pass me by, but it stops to
see me cry.
So painful and sad, sometimes I cry and no one cares about why,
Except Caroline.

"Just a poem to you that I wrote to show you what an impact you have made on my life. I thank you for your compassion and whether or not I succeed, I will remember you always. But, I WILL succeed. Have faith in me. From an adopted Grandson, Ramone, 2001."

(Ramone was a patient on one of the units in which I worked. He is not related to me and I have never seen him again. I can only assume and pray that he has succeeded in his life.)

CHAPTER 2

NURSING EDUCATION: UNIVERSITY OF MINNESOTA

Pre-Nursing: University of Minnesota

We did not have a counselor in my high school, so the principal, Mr. Thompson, took on that role. He did not think I should go to school in the "big city," so he would not help me. He suggested that I attend a three-year hospital-based nursing school closer to home, since all my friends were doing this. Or better yet, he said I could become a secretary, because I "would just get married anyway and already knew how to type."

So, I had to fill out all the papers for admission to the U myself.

I even got a scholarship, which Thompson had to present to me at graduation. (The University of Minnesota currently has over 35,000 undergraduate students and over 12,500 graduate students. The several campuses include Minneapolis, St. Paul, Duluth, Morris, Rochester, and Crookston.)

A virtual graduation was held in May of 2020 with about 17,000 graduates.

Sanford Hall

My freshman year at the University, I lived in Sanford Hall, the first women's dormitory on campus, having been built in 1910.

It was named for Professor Maria Sanford (1836-1920), an American educator and national advocate for women's rights. She was one of the first women in the U.S. to be named to a college professorship. A number of facilities throughout the US are named for Sanford, including a World War II Liberty Ship, the *SS Maria Sanford*. (Adapted from *Maria Sanford Biography* – Wikipedia)

While living in Sanford Hall, I met some other pre-nursing students, who have become my life-long friends.

Dress-Up Evenings

On Wednesday evenings, we were required to wear dresses and nice shoes to dinner in the dorm. If we did not do so, we were not allowed to enter the dining room. One time, my roommate Barb, had her pajamas on. She rolled up the cuffs and wore a long coat. Just after she entered the dining room, the pajama legs began to unroll, so she got caught and was not allowed to eat that evening. Clothing choices in college today are certainly MUCH different.

Food Poisoning in the Dormitory

Just before Christmas, we had a big buffet. Of the more than 300 girls in the dorm, all but about six, became ill with food poisoning after the buffet. There was no way to identify the offending food, since there were so many choices. I have no idea why I didn't get sick, but I didn't. At first, they took the sickest girls to the hospital, some of whom even had seizures.

They soon realized that too many people were sick and the hospital did not have room, so they set up an *infirmary in the dorm*. We had nurses and a doctor in the dormitory around the clock. Since I wasn't sick, I was drafted to help pass out medications, take temperatures, and monitor the girls. We had a cart and made rounds in the dorm, passing out anti-emetics (to prevent vomiting), anti-diarrheals (to treat diarrhea), and other comfort medications, such as aspirin and Tylenol, (which was very new at that time, having begun use in 1955.)

However, since this occurred during finals week and I was not sick,

I also had to take my final examinations. So, by a quirk of fate, *I began my actual nursing career in college during my first quarter.*

The Car Accident

My best friend from high school, Betty, also lived in Sanford Hall. One evening, as she was crossing University Avenue, she was struck by a car. She was quite badly injured, lost some teeth, and had permanent paralysis of part of her face. I was summoned to administer First Aid until the police got there.

This incident did not hold her back, however. Several years later, Betty was runner-up to the Minneapolis Aquatennial Queen! (She remained one of my best friends until her death in 2018.)

And, again I was doing nursing duties before entering nursing school.

Zoology

Nursing students were required to take a two-quarter course in Zoology. You had to pass the first quarter in order to continue on into the second quarter. This course was very difficult and many students did not make it through. After taking the final examination for the first quarter, we knew the scores would be posted in the Zoology building, but we would not be able to see them until the next day.

We were so worried that we forced open a window in the building; that is, we "broke in," so we could see our scores that evening. All my best friends passed, as did I. And fortunately, we did not get caught.

The Lobster Dinner

During the Zoology class, we had to dissect a lobster (ish.) One night, a group of us went out to dinner and a Pre-Med student named Dave ordered lobster. Then, he proceeded to dissect it and identify each structure as he ate it. Some of us lost our appetites.

Chemistry

We also had to take chemistry as a prerequisite for nursing. Because of scheduling conflicts, I ended up in the chemistry class with the chemistry majors and pre-med students. The professor (Dr. Brastad) was amazing. He would lecture about one thing, while writing another thing on the board. We were forced to team up. One student would write everything he said and the other would write what was on the board. And, amazingly these two things came together and made sense. I will never know how the professor did this.

We were required to memorize many formulas, and we were allowed to use a *slide rule*. (There were no calculators then.) I had never used a slide rule and could not figure it out. I could do the mathematical calculations and formulas the long way (in my head or on paper), but it took a lot of time.

I talked to the professor and we made a deal. He assigned a student assistant to monitor me when we had an exam. Since this class was the last one of the day, I could stay as long as I needed to and the monitor had to stay with me while I figured out all the formulas longhand. I brought supper for both of us. I passed the course, but it was really difficult.

Swimming

We had to take a certain number of Physical Education courses. I took swimming during the very cold winter. Usually, it was about zero or below by the time I got out of the pool. So, instead of drying my hair, I would just go back to the dorm. However, on very cold days my hair would be frozen by the time I got home. It's a wonder I didn't die of pneumonia!

But that's nothing. On February 2, 1996, I was snowmobiling with a bunch of guys in Tower, Minnesota, when the all-time low temperature record for the state was set. It was *sixty below zero, actual temperature, not wind chill!* (We waited until it was forty below zero before we started riding.)

Since I was the only woman, I didn't say anything. Tough nurse!

SPECIAL SITUATIONS

The University Football Band

I was a member of the Band during my first two years at the U. At that time, women were not allowed to march on the football field, but we did many tasks. We played from the sidelines for football games and we played in Pep Bands for basketball and hockey games. When students first started in band, they were called "Stooges" for the first week and were given tasks by the "Veterans."

The week before my freshman year started, I was a Stooge. Many high school bands from all over Minnesota were invited to "Band Day." They arrived in school buses, my high school among them. Since I had only been out of high school for a couple months, I knew all the Sauk Centre students.

My Stooge task on Band Day was to stand in the middle of Washington Avenue in Minneapolis and tell the buses where to go. It was raining and I was wearing a floor-length dark-colored coat. It's a wonder the bus drivers could even see me. Someone must have called my mother and told her.

That night I received a frantic call. My mother said, "Were you really directing traffic in Minneapolis?" (So much for relaxing and not worrying about your little daughter alone in the big city!)

When I entered the School of Nursing, I was told I could no longer be in the band, because I wouldn't have time. So, I was required to choose between nursing and the band. Fortunately, I chose nursing. (Today, there are several nursing students in the Band, as well as a football player.)

Twenty years later, at the age of thirty-eight, I marched as a regular member of the Marching Band. (Chapter 6)

The Auschwitz Escape

While living in Sanford Hall, Gretchen, a Jewish girl from Germany, told us about her memories of World War II. When she was about six, she and her parents were on one of the trains bound for Auschwitz

Concentration Camp. The train stopped for water near some woods and many people jumped off, amid gunshots.

She and her mother crawled and ran through the weeds into the woods and hid. They eventually made it to Minnesota. They escaped sure death in Auschwitz, but sadly, her father was lost. (We in the United States were pretty much uninformed as to what was happening in Europe.)

Grabbed on the Sidewalk

I had taken Red Cross Swimming and Lifesaving classes prior to coming to the U. In my second year at the U, I lived in a sorority house on a side street where it was quite dark. (I was very small at that time.)

I was walking home one evening and suddenly I was grabbed around the neck from behind. Without thinking, I used my Red Cross training to break the hold and flip the guy onto his back. I took off running and left him lying on the ground. I am sure he had no idea what had happened to him. Big surprise! After that, I tried always to walk with someone else, but I felt that my Red Cross training had possibly saved my life.

Later, when I worked on Psych/Mental Health, I learned this and many other self-defense procedures. (Chapter 12)

Fortunately, I have never had to use these again.

Associate in Liberal Arts Degree

My second year in college, a friend said if I took one more course in Spanish, I could get a two year degree. (I had already taken three quarters of Spanish.) This seemed like a good idea, so I did it. My father was able to see me receive my two-year degree in June of 1957 before he died.

I received an ALA degree. (Associate in Liberal Arts)

My major was pre-nursing.

At that time, there were no junior colleges and very few people had ever heard of an Associate Degree, particularly from the University. There were no two-year nursing programs. (General College at the U did offer an AA degree in general education.)

My ALA degree later served to get me a job at Burke Marketing Research while I was in college. (Chapter 10)

This job helped me make some money for college and also enabled me to meet and talk with people of all socioeconomic groups. This proved to be very valuable in my nursing career and in my future life.

CLA Graduation and "Probiehood"

In 1957, a mass ceremony was held for everyone graduating from the entire University. All the graduates (about 6,000) were honored together, which was held in the open-air Memorial Stadium. We marched in as fast as people could walk, because it was threatening to rain.

After marching in, I took my place in the band. My father later said, "It was a really good thing you were in the band, because otherwise, I would never have been able to pick you out of that huge crowd."

After two years of college, we had to reapply for admission to the School of Nursing. (A number of my classmates went to other colleges the first two years. And a number of pre-nursing students didn't get accepted into the School of Nursing.)

During the first two quarters of the actual nursing program, we were known as "probies" (probationers) until we were "capped." Then, we could wear our nursing student caps and uniforms and were officially nursing students.

Today, the University has a "guaranteed acceptance" plan. Some nursing students are admitted as freshmen and are guaranteed to be accepted into the nursing program after their basic courses. This takes much of the pressure off and allows these students to relax and concentrate on their required courses.

I have not heard of any of these students who did not study and receive the required grades in the pre-nursing portion of the program.

Basic Nursing Skills

During the two-quarter probationary period, we were taught basic nursing skills such as giving bed baths, making hospital beds, and measuring vital signs (temperature, pulse, respiration, and blood pressure.)

Frequent handwashing was emphasized. We were taught to sing "Yankee Doodle" or "Happy Birthday" (twice) while doing handwashing (about twenty seconds.) This is still the recommended length of time for a thorough handwash. We were also taught to give patients a partial sponge bath. Among the students this was called a "PTA bath." ("Pits, Tits, and A—")

Currently, additional emphasis is being placed on frequent handwashing. Several years ago, before the COVID-19 virus scare, my daughter-in-law, who is a nurse, was washing her hands in a public rest room. Another lady came up to her and said, "You must be a nurse. You were humming 'Yankee Doodle.'"

Nursing Capping

Receiving the nursing cap in a special ceremony was a big event in the life of all nursing students at that time. Our student caps were traditional nurses' caps, with "wings" which stuck out. I was especially happy about capping, because my father was able to be there. He passed away before I graduated from the nursing program.

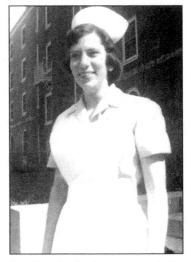

University of Minnesota School of Nursing

(This portion of this chapter is dedicated to my roommate and confidant Judy. We had these adventures together and are still good friends.)

Caroline Bunker's capping photo, showing the University of Minnesota student nursing cap, March 1958 (BHMedia)

The Nursing School at the University of Minnesota was originally founded in 1909.

Isabel Hampton Robb of Johns Hopkins convinced Dr. Richard Olding Beard that there should be a nursing program at the collegiate level somewhere in the United States; Minnesota was chosen.

The program was originally called the "University of Minnesota School for Nurses."

The first "Superintendent of Nurses" was Bertha Erdman, who became ill and resigned after one year.

Katherine Jane Densford (Dreeves)

The Director of the School of Nursing from 1930 to 1959 was Miss Katherine Densford. She was very proper and professional. She was born in 1890 and had degrees in History and Latin and later earned a Masters' Degree. (She was ahead of her time, because most women did not go to college then, particularly to Graduate School.)

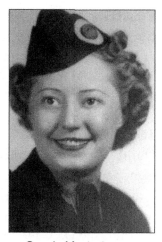

Cousin Mavis Amman (Rondeau), Nursing Cadet, World War II (WWII or WW2), also known as the Second World War, was a global war that lasted from 1939 to 1945 (Photo courtesy of Judy Milam)

As a result of World War I, she then pursued nursing at the School of Nursing and Health in Cincinnati. She became an expert in Public Health and tuberculosis ("TB", also known as "consumption.")

At that time many patients, as well as nurses, died of TB. This inspired Miss Densford to include a TB rotation in our program. This was probably the only one, or one of very few, nursing programs to have such a rotation.

Miss Densford received many honors, including the Presidency of important national and international nursing organizations. The International Center for Nursing Leadership at the University of Minnesota is named for her, as is the Weaver/Densford building. We were very fortunate to have her as our Director.

(Information from *Katherine Densford Dreeves: Marching at the Head of the Parade*, PhD Thesis by Lauren Kay Glass, University of Minnesota, 1988)

Kimi Hara

Kimi Hara was a Japanese woman who was placed in a "confinement camp" in California during World War II. Somehow, Densford learned about her and rescued her from the camp. Hara was brought to Minnesota where she became a leader in nursing.

The Cadet Program

During World War II, there was a great need for nurses and the government announced that nurses would be drafted into the Army. Densford made a deal with the government, saying she would train nurses quickly to avoid having them drafted.

Thus, the US Cadet Nurse Corps was born and hundreds of nurses were trained at the University of Minnesota, the largest number trained anywhere. This became the model for all Cadet Programs in the US and many hospitals and colleges were involved. The need for nurses was met and the draft was not necessary, thanks to Densford. (Two of my husband's cousins were nursing cadets at the University of Minnesota.)

Nursing College Board and Alumni Board

As a student, I was a member of the Nursing College Board (NCB), made up of students, faculty, and Miss Densford. This was a great honor. Miss Densford was very serious and formal and had a slight British-type accent. She had never married.

Densford retired during my last year in school (at the end of 1959.) A small party was held for her by the NCB. At the party, she stood up and quietly said, "I am being married this afternoon and this evening we are going to Europe," and then she sat down. You could have heard a pin drop. Only one faculty member knew she had a "boy friend" (Mr. Dreeves.) We were all astounded. (She was married at the age of 69. She and Dreeves were married for more than eighteen years before her death in 1978.)

About ten years after I graduated, I was at the office of the Minnesota Board of Nursing and Ms. Densford-Dreeves saw me and said, "I remember you. You are Caroline Bunker and you graduated in 1959 or '60."

I was amazed that she remembered me by name and when I graduated.

After graduation, I served several terms on the Alumni Board of Trustees for the School of Nursing. In addition, I was the liaison to the Nursing Foundation. I have assisted in events such as the Annual Spring Celebration and the Jewelry Sale for nursing scholarships. I have also been involved in activities for the School such as speed mentoring, resume' evaluation, and practice job interviews.

The Nursing Program Today

The University of Minnesota Nursing Program has had only ten directors in its more than 100 years.

The current Dean is Connie White Delaney (since 2005.)

The school is exceptional and is ranked very highly in the country.

Today there are nearly 900 graduate and undergraduate students in the school. (U of M information, Google, 2019)

The "New" Football Stadium

One day in 2009, a senior nursing student called me and said the school had given her my name. She was to interview me about my life as a nurse. She did not have a car, so I said I would meet her on campus. I have been involved with the U Band for many years and we had a meeting scheduled in the *brand new TCF Bank Stadium*, which had just been built. I told her I had a meeting on campus in a few days and she asked where. I told her it was in the stadium and she was astounded. "Really? The new stadium? Oh, my goodness!"

She was so impressed that I could do no wrong after that!

The 100 Distinguished Alumni Award

In 2009, for the 100th anniversary of the School of Nursing, I was fortunate enough to be named as one of "100 Distinguished Alumni," *an award which has been given only once in the history of the School.*

This was a great honor. (And, our photos are permanently displayed in the lobby of the Weaver-Densford Building.)

My husband and several of my friends attended the dinner and the Centennial ceremony.

The description in the Centennial Celebration Program for the event stated:

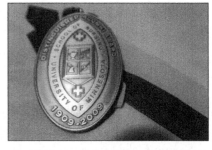

Rosdahl was named one of 100 "Distinguished Alumni" of the Minnesota School of Nursing Centennial, 2009—Shown here is the medal awarded (CB Rosdahl)

CAROLINE BUNKER ROSDAHL, 1960

"Recognized for her contributions as the Director of a Public Health Nursing Service responsible for healthcare within industry, nursing homes, and school settings. She mentored high school students to encourage their pursuit of health careers and developed the initial nursing

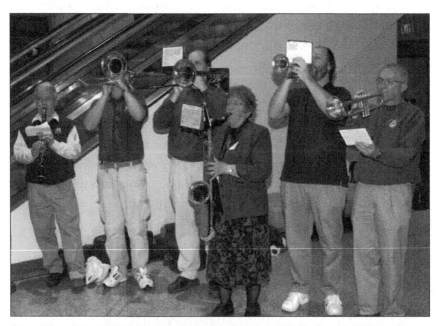

Rosdahl and the Minnesota Alumni Band playing at the Centennial Award Dinner (Keith Bunker Rosdahl)

curriculum along with other health related programs within a technical college setting. Her landmark book, *Textbook of Basic Nursing*, is in its ninth edition and is widely used throughout the world."

A few days before the award ceremony, an official from the School of Nursing called and asked if I could provide a band to play at the dinner. So, I gathered some of my friends from the Alumni Band and we entertained the dinner guests. Being in the Band came in handy again. And now it was OK with the School of Nursing that I was in the Band!

Powell Hall

While we were nursing students, we worked thirty hours a week in the hospital, in exchange for room and board. I would never have been able to go to college without this. (The practice of earning room and board was discontinued soon after we were there.)

After capping, all nursing students were required to live in the nursing dormitory (Powell Hall), unless they were married. Living there was a big advantage for us, in addition to the fact that it was free. In Powell Hall, we lived together, ate together, and worked together.

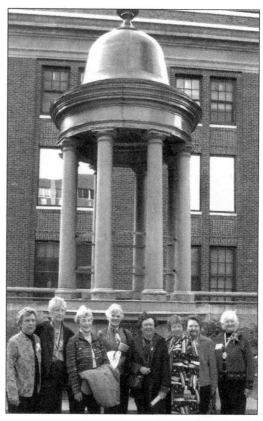

Powell Hall cupola with representatives of the Nursing Class of 1960 (BH Media)

We had "rotation groups" of about eight students and we rotated through the clinical specialties together. Most rotations were about three months long. Therefore, we became very close friends. Many of us still see each other, 60+ years later. (Today, nursing students live in apartments, other dormitories, or their own homes. They do not have nearly the camaraderie that we had.)

Powell Hall was built in 1932 and named for Louise Powell, Superintendent of Nurses from 1910 to 1924. It was torn down in 1981, after nearly fifty years of occupancy, to make way for new medical facilities.

The cupola from Powell Hall now stands proudly on the lawn in front of the former location of the dorm. The House Mother of Powell Hall when we were students was Mrs. Hayes. She was the widow of a pastor in my home town, so I knew her quite well. More about that later . . . .

(Information from *History of Our School Leadership*, 2019, Regents of the University of Minnesota. Wikipedia)

DORMITORY STORIES

The Doorknob

Since Powell Hall was an old building, it had an old elevator. In order to enter the elevator, you grasped a fancy brass doorknob and pulled a solid door toward you. Then, you slid an inner folding gate sideways to the right.

One day, the doorknob fell off and the manager of the dorm called the Otis Elevator Company for repairs. The people at the company said, "Our elevators don't have doorknobs." They were informed that this Otis elevator did indeed have a doorknob.

The company sent about ten people out to do the repair, because they all wanted to see an Otis elevator with a doorknob.

The Antlers

My roommate was a camper and outdoorswoman. She brought home a set of deer antlers she had found in the North Woods and these were displayed in our Powell Hall dorm room. We had a little tiny housekeeper with a very high voice and bright red dyed hair—Minnie.

24

She was afraid of the antlers. So, she would just throw the bed sheets into our room and would not come in.

Nearly twenty years later, I was in the Marching Band at the University. (Chapter 6)

We marched and played a concert in downtown Minneapolis. After the concert, little Minnie came up to me and said, "I remember you. You're the one with the antlers!"

The Dye Job

One day, one of the girls in the dorm decided to dye her hair black. She used the laundry room sink to do this and *huge permanent black stains* were left on the sink. The next day, there was a sign, presumably written by Minnie, that said, "Don't *die* in here."

High Jinks in Dorm Rooms

One of the men's dormitories named Pioneer Hall was a block away from Powell Hall. One week-end, a male student went home and left his old Model-T car at the U (bad idea.) A bunch of us took it apart, piece by piece, and reassembled it in his room. It totally filled his dorm room. (Remember: this was the 1950s; girls were not allowed in the men's dorm.) Of course, the car had to be taken apart again to get it back down to the street.

Another time, someone got a huge weather balloon. We took it up to a guy's third floor dorm room and filled it with water from the fire hose. When the door was opened, the balloon would bulge out the door. There was only one tiny problem—we hadn't planned a way to let the water out of the balloon without flooding the dorm.

So, someone got the brilliant idea to have a guy *climb up the outside of the building*, open the window and stab the balloon, allowing the water to drain outside. I was stationed on the corner as a lookout. As I was standing there, the House Mother from Powell Hall, Mrs. Hayes, approached. (Remember, I knew her well from my home town.) I knew the water was going to come down soon, but I didn't dare move because I didn't want to give away the secret.

So, as we were standing there, a huge flood of water came cascading down on us. She just looked up at the guy hanging on the side of the building, at the water rushing down the side of the building, and at me. And she said, "You knew about this didn't you?"

I can't believe we didn't get in trouble, but we had some fun in addition to our nursing studies. Today, dorms are often co-ed, so men and women live in the same dorm. It would not be nearly as exciting now, because women are not forbidden to be in the "men's" dorm.

Selected Nursing Care Studies

We were assigned care studies on nearly every rotation. We were to carefully research the case, write up a report, and present our findings to the class. We became friends with most of our care study patients.

Susan B—Patent Ductus Arteriosis

Susan was a young girl brought to the University Hospital from Milwaukee for repair of a *patent ductus arteriosus* (PDA) because the University was a pioneer in heart surgery. (The ductus is a vessel *exterior to the heart*. This vessel connects the aorta [*carrying oxygenated blood to the entire body*] and the pulmonary artery [*carrying unoxygenated blood to the lungs*].) The ductus should close at birth, but Susan's was still open [*patent*].)

At that time, repair of a patent ductus involved opening the chest. This repair was considered to be major heart surgery. It was very difficult and dangerous, even though the heart did not need to be stopped and no incision was made into the heart itself. Susan's surgery was successful and she recovered completely.

Today, this surgery is done with a very small chest incision (called a "stab wound") or may actually be done by entering through the blood vessels. In some cases, a small patent ductus closes spontaneously.

Gabriel P—Heart Surgery

We also had a young boy, Gabriel, who was flown in from Mexico for open heart surgery, which was quite experimental at that time. Mexico did not have the facilities to perform the procedure. Since the U of M was noted for heart surgery, Gabriel came there. The procedure went well and Gabriel returned home to a much better life.

Marc S—The Boy in a Bubble

Marc was a teen-age boy brought to Minnesota from Eastern Europe for treatment. He had a non-functioning immune system for which there were no medications at that time. He was the proverbial "boy in a bubble" that we had heard about.

With recent concern about COVID-19, a device patterned after the "bubble" is now sometimes being used. (Its formal name is the *biohazard or biological containment unit.*)

Marc was older than most children with his disorder (*agammaglobulinemia*), because these children are lacking the mechanisms for immunity and usually die in early childhood. They are very prone to life-threatening infections. We cared for Marc by actually going inside the bubble. We wore sterile surgical gowns and gloves, with surgical caps and masks.

This is much like the nurses of today, except we were trying to protect the patient from any dangerous (*pathogenic*) organisms we might be carrying. Today, nurses are wearing protective gear to protect themselves from pathogens the patient might have and to prevent spreading them to other patients.

Caring for Marc was an amazing experience. We felt sorry for him. I don't know what happened to him, but if he lived long enough, he would probably have been able to function outside the bubble with the aid of antiviral medications and gamma globulin, as well as protective gear developed later.

John M—The Polio Victim

John was a young man only about two years younger than I. He was transferred in for rehabilitation from Nebraska, where his mother was an important legislator. He was one of the last people to get paralyzing polio (*poliomyelitis*) before immunizations to prevent it became available.

He was basically paralyzed from the chest down, although he was able to talk and breathe on his own and to do some things with his arms, hands, and fingers in slings. He ran his motorized wheelchair with head movements.

I stayed in touch with John for years after he left the hospital. John was a brilliant and amazing young man. He got a PhD in physics and math and taught at the University of California. He was also a wine expert and taught classes in colleges and for the vineyards.

In addition, John invented a number of assistive items for disabled people and holds many patents. He was a wonderful model for people with disabilities. John married one of his caregivers, but I don't think they had children. He made himself a good life, despite his disability. John would now be in his late seventies or early eighties.

The Iron Lung

As students, we were taught how to pump an "Iron Lung," in case the electrical power went out. This was a large mechanical machine, which simulated the negative pressure in the chest, causing breathing.

The person who was paralyzed and could not breathe without assistance was placed in the machine, which enclosed his/her entire body except the head.

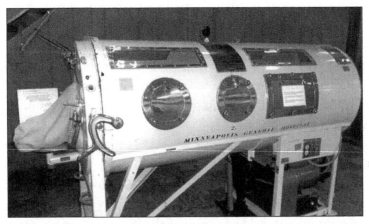

The Iron Lung saved many lives during the polio epidemics of the 1940s and 1950s (CB Rosdahl and Minneapolis General Hospital)

Patients lived in the "lung" and were cared for through special arm/hand openings.

The iron lung saved many lives and was used extensively during the polio epidemics of the 1940s and '50s.

The Level One Trauma Hospital in Minneapolis has an iron lung on display and I amazed my coworkers (in about 2000) by demonstrating how it worked. These young nurses had never heard of, seen, or used, an iron lung.

External mechanical ventilators are now used to maintain respiration and, for example, are being used to care for severe cases of COVID-19.

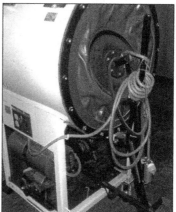

The Iron Lung could be pumped manually, in case of a power failure (CB Rosdahl)

Medical-Surgical Nursing (MED-SURG)

We cared for people with many serious disorders while we were students on Medical-Surgical units. Often, patients were transferred to the University because their local hospital could not handle the severity of their cases.

My Dying Friend

A man from my hometown, Lawrence B, was in the hospital. He had a son my age and they went to my church, so I knew him very well. He was terminally ill. I went to see him and he obviously wanted to talk to me about his impending death, but his wife would not allow this and would not leave the room. I still think of this and feel badly, because maybe I could have helped him by allowing him to express his feelings.

The D and E Girl

One assignment for Med-Surg students was to be the "D and E Girl."

This stood for *douche and enema.*

The assignment was to go around very early in the morning and administer douches and enemas, one after another, all morning. This was definitely not the favorite assignment for students!

The Autopsy

We were required to observe at least one autopsy (post-mortem examination) while we were students. The one that I observed was a young single girl who had tried to induce an abortion by taking a large dose of quinine. (Medical abortions were illegal at that time.) At autopsy, it was discovered that she *had never been pregnant*. So, it was an unnecessary death and very sad. This is the only autopsy I have ever observed.

The Stool Sample Refrigerator

There was a special refrigerator on Med-Surg designated by a big sign, "For Stools Only." When we came to that unit on our first day, the Instructor was showing us around. She opened the refrigerator door and inside stood a *bedside step stool* from one of the patient rooms. (My roommate's boyfriend was an orderly and we all knew he had put it there, but he didn't get caught.) We thought it was very funny; our instructor was not amused.

The Light-Skinned Black Nurse

One of the head nurses was a very light-skinned mixed-race woman. Mixed-race people were very rare in those days. This nurse was very pretty and bright. However, she told us she had problems dating. In those days, mixed-race marriages were almost nonexistent. Black men would not go out with her, because she looked white. And, often they did not believe she was mixed-race. In addition, she didn't feel she could go with a white man because she didn't want to misrepresent herself, even though she could easily have passed. She was also fearful she might have a black child. As far as I know, she never married.

Operating Room (OR): The Surgeons

We were very fortunate to be able to participate in groundbreaking surgical procedures as part of our nursing education. Many of these

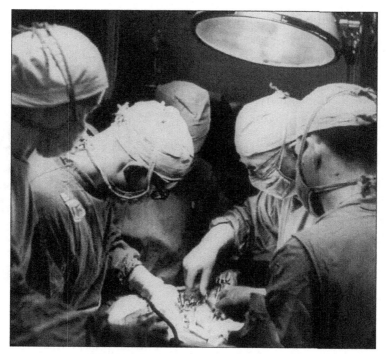

A typical Operating Room scene, 1950s

procedures were the basis for more advanced techniques still used today.

Dr. C. Walton Lillehei

The OR was a major adventure. We spent about three months there and I loved it.

We were definitely "trained on-the-job," but we learned a lot. We "scrubbed-in" (to assist in surgery) for several very famous surgeons.

One of these men was Dr. C. Walton Lillehei (1918-1999), who "pioneered open-heart surgery, as well as numerous techniques, equipment and prostheses for cardiothoracic surgery." (Wikipedia)

His Operating Room was designated as "Room J."

Lillehei wrote several books and won a number of awards, including the Bronze Star for World War ll service. He was inducted into the Minnesota Inventors Hall of Fame in 1993. In 1966-'67, he was

President of the American College of Cardiology. (U of Minnesota Information Service)

Lillehei was known as "*the father of open-heart surgery*." He assisted in the very first open-heart surgery performed by F. John Lewis. People came to the U from all over the world to learn procedures and/or to have heart surgery.

In 1954, the "heart-lung" machine ("bubble oxygenator") was developed and allowed *open-heart procedures* to be done. (American Heart Association Journal, 1999)

Dr. Lillehei died in 1999 at the age of eighty. The Lillehei Heart Institute at the University of Minnesota carries his name. Lillehei's "*manual dexterity was developed in his youth by repairing his Model-T Ford.*" (From an article in a medical journal)

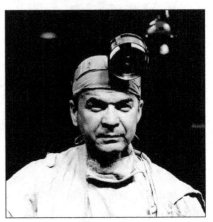

Dr. C. Walton Lillehei, known as "the Father of Open-Heart Surgery" (University of Minnesota Libraries, University Archives)

Lillehei's wife, Katherine ("Kaye"), a graduate of the University's nursing program, was very active in the U of Minnesota Nursing Alumni Association. She died in 2012. I was there when she "landed the first blow" to demolish a wall for a new nursing laboratory.

Dr. Owen H. Wangensteen

Dr. Wangensteen (1898-1981), during my time at the University in the late 1950s, was Chief of Surgery. He was particularly known for his remarkable memory. He "began his medical practice in caring for the animals on the farm. He is thought to have been the first in his county to vaccinate for anthrax." (Wangensteen Historical Library)

Wangensteen developed the Wangensteen tube, "which used suction to treat small bowel obstruction, an innovation estimated to have saved a million lives by the time of his death." (Wikipedia)

Wangensteen Suction

Wangensteen suction, invented by Dr. W, was used throughout the U hospital. It was very effective, but cumbersome. It consisted of three large one-gallon bottles, one of which was filled with water and held up on an IV pole in a cloth sling. As water flowed into a lower bottle, a gentle suction was created. A third bottle collected drainage.

The major problem with this suction was refilling and managing the upper bottle. Sometimes the plug came out and you had water all over. And if you dropped a bottle, at the very least you had water all over and in the worst case, you

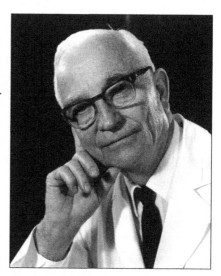

Dr. Owen H. Wangensteen, the inventor of Wangensteen suction, which saved thousands of lives (Wangensteen Historical Library, University Archives, University of Minnesota Libraries)

had broken glass AND water all over. Wangensteen suction was used at the U long after mechanical suction became available, because of Dr. W.

In the TV show, M.A.S.H., "Colonel Potter" set up and explained the suction when they lost power. He used a pickle bottle and a mustard bottle and it was repaired in the next episode. (Season 8, Episodes 4 and 5)

Potter identified Dr. Wangensteen by name (although he pronounced the name wrong.)

I am probably one of a very few nurses now who has ever worked with this device and knew what it was.

The M.A.S.H. doctors also rigged up a device for defibrillation of the heart in another episode. (Season 10, Episode 19)

And, in another episode, a special vascular (blood vessel) clamp, which is still used today, was developed. (Season 6, Episode 17)

Dr. Wangensteen once said: "In summary, plant a tree for posterity in the orchard of your profession. It will give you enduring satisfaction, though you may never live to see it mature; its growth can project your image and wishes far into time and space." (In the *Journal of the American Medical Association,* 1968; quoted in Buchwald, Page 153—see Bibliography)

Other Famous Surgeons
I met a number of other surgeons who did record-breaking work.

Wangensteen had been a mentor to Lillehei and a number of these other famous surgeons.

Richard Varco (1913-2004) was noted for helping "perform the first successful open heart and obesity operations." On September 2, 1952, Dr. Varco and his colleagues at the University of Minnesota performed the first successful operation on a beating human heart, saving a five-year-old girl who had been born with a heart murmur. Until then, surgeons had found it impossible to perform open cardiac procedures, because the heart pulsated with blood. The team, led by Dr. C. Walton Lillehei . . .used a risky technique (super-cooling the patient, to slow the heart) that had worked on animals." (New York Times, 5-12-1994)

Another famous surgeon Christiaan Barnard (1922-2001), came from South Africa to study at the University of Minnesota. In 1956, he performed his first heart surgery and in 1967, he performed his first heart transplant. He originally intended to be a general surgeon, but became fascinated by heart surgery at Minnesota. (Google, 2019)

Dr. Harvey Buchwald came to the University just after I graduated. He was known as a "pioneer of metabolic and bariatric (obesity) surgery." He is the holder of the "Wangensteen Chair in Experimental Surgery (Emeritus)" at the U. (American College of Surgeons and Wikipedia, 2020)

Buchwald has just written a book, *Surgical Renaissance in the Heartland . . . a Memoir of the Wangensteen Era.* (See Bibliography)

When one of these noted surgeons was operating, you could almost see the red carpet and hear the trumpets playing as they entered the room. We were so fortunate to have the opportunity to scrub for them.

Adventures in the Operating Room

Heart Surgery: Dr. Lillehei and Judy

It was our *very first day in the operating room* as students. We had almost NO previous orientation to the Operating Room (OR). Dr. Lillehei was doing an open-heart procedure, which involved stopping the heart and using the heart-lung machine (pump oxygenator, "bubble oxygenator") to circulate blood through the body. This was very new technology and was very precarious.

Judy, my roommate, was "scrubbed in" for the surgery (assisting the surgeon.)

Dr. Lillehei said to her, "Now when I tell you, clamp that blood vessel."

So, when he said so, she clamped the blood vessel.

She later realized that this was the *aorta, the largest blood vessel in the body*, which comes directly out of the heart and carries blood to the entire body. And, this was her *first day in the OR!* So, she clamped the vessel and the surgery was successful. We were so young and innocent. She didn't have time to be afraid.

The Book

I have the First Edition of a special book, *The Operation—A Minute-by-Minute Account of a Heart Operation*. (See Bibliography)

The book is signed, "To Caroline Bunker—with my best wishes. C. Walton Lillehei MD, Dec. 1958."

It is also signed by the Head Nurse in Room J (the Heart Surgery OR), Miss Clara Monroe RN:

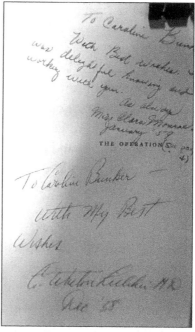

Signatures in the book: *The Operation . . . a minute-by-minute account of a heart operation* (CB Rosdahl)

35

"To Caroline Bunker. With best wishes. It was delightful knowing and working with you."

Another signature is from Jim Wade, the CV (Cardiovascular) Technician. He was the expert in running the heart-lung oxygenator (bubble oxygenator). He drew a blue star and then wrote, "This blue star should have been put on your record, the one I make for goodies in Room J. See you later in J."

Another complimentary inscription is in Spanish, from P. Aguierre, a visiting surgeon from Mexico.

Dr. Wangensteen's Stool

Dr. W. was not a tall man, so he had to stand on a special stool in order to reach the operative area. One staff person was always assigned to move this stool from place to place for him. And, the staff called the stool "God's Little Acre."

Of course, he did not know this.

The Fish Tank

One of the famous surgeons had a deep stainless steel tank, filled with zephiran, in the operating room (OR).

Zephiran (benzalkonium chloride) is a disinfectant solution, but is not sterile. The surgeon would do the careful surgical scrub of his hands and forearms and then dip into the zephiran tank.

This basically *defeated the purpose* of the surgical scrub. Everyone knew this, but nobody was brave enough to say anything, because he was so important.

But, we dopey students were indestructible. So, one night Judy and I sneaked into the OR, dumped out the zephiran, and replaced it with water and goldfish. The next day, the surgeon did his scrub, walked into the OR, and bent over to dip into the tank. He stopped and stared.

When he saw the fish swimming around, he turned and went directly to the OR table to begin the procedure. He did not say a word and neither did anyone else, but he never used the tank again. And, nobody ever knew who had done the zephiran/water switch.

"Whoops!

One day, one of the most famous surgeons was operating and he accidentally severed the patient's ureter (the tube from the kidney to the bladder.) The only thing he said was "Whoops!" At that time, there was no way to repair the damage, so the patient's kidney had to be removed.

I don't know, but I might guess that the surgeon went out to the patient's family and said, "When we got in there, we found that one of his kidneys was diseased, so we had to remove it."

We will never know. (The patient, of course, was able to live a normal life with only one kidney.)

Kidney Transplant Recipient

An aside. One of my friends, Connie, is one of the oldest living kidney transplant recipients in the country. (In 2020, she will be *forty-eight years post-transplant.*)

She worked at the University, but her surgery was done at the Mayo Clinic in Rochester. The surgeons at the University always felt badly, because they would have liked to use her case as an example.

Halloween and Dr. French

One Halloween day I was assigned to Neurosurgery.

Dr. Lyle French (1915-2004) was a famous neurosurgeon. That day, he was doing an open-skull procedure. The patient was awake, to enable him to respond to commands.

In preparation for the surgery, the patient's head was shaved and painted with the orange prep solution used in all surgeries. Dr. French then took his magic marker, as always, to indicate where incisions and burr holes were to be made.

However, instead of this, he drew a Jack-O-Lantern face on the patient's orange skull. Now, remember, the patient was awake, so we could not laugh.

PS: Dr. French performed brain surgery on my mother who had metastatic (spreading) cancer. He was unable to do anything to help her. He did not send a bill, so I asked him about it.

He said, "I know your mother was a teacher and I know she didn't have any money. I was not able to help her, so there will be no charge."

He finally agreed to accept whatever her insurance would pay, but no more.

French was a wonderful man. After I left the U, he ran dogs with me in field trials, so I got to know him personally. In addition, he shared an office with Jane, one of my good friends, and she liked him very much.

The Flying Operating Room Light

In each OR, there was a huge light mounted on a track in the ceiling over the operating table. Surgery that day was to be performed on a very famous man, so an important and renowned surgeon had been brought in from another university to perform this delicate surgery. Everyone was nervous about having this famous guest surgeon coming in. The tension in the OR was more palpable than usual that day.

One of my classmates was circulating in the OR (not scrubbed in.) The famous surgeon said to her, "Could you adjust that light a little?" She gave it a big shove; it flew down the track, hit the surgeon on the head, and knocked him out!

He was lying on the floor of the OR on his back and everyone was absolutely panicky.

When he came to, he quietly said, "Maybe not quite that much."

Heating Up Pizza

One night we had a pizza that had gotten cold. Since there were no microwaves in those days, we decided to use the autoclave (sterilizer) in the Operating Room area to heat it up. The only problem was that the autoclave was vented throughout the entire hospital, which we didn't know. The place smelled like Dominos for several days. Of course, nobody knew why. And nobody knew who did it.

Pediatrics (PEDS)

Here is where Marc, Susan, and Gabriel were my care studies. There were many other stories during this rotation. I remember one little toddler who had a severe heart defect. He was very *cyanotic* (blue). And, he had a *pink pacifier* in his mouth all the time as he toddled around the unit. The combination of the pink pacifier and the blue mouth was really outstanding. That turned me off pacifiers forever.

We did many heart surgeries, working with the surgeons mentioned above.

These surgeries were often like miracles, because the children were so limited before the procedure. After the procedure, many of them were able to live normal lives.

Pediatrics could also be very sad, because most of the patients at the University were critically ill and had been transferred from other hospitals. We did not often see common ailments or simple surgeries, unless the parents were students or professors at the school. Everything was difficult and complex. But, many lives were saved that would not have been saved at other hospitals.

Obstetrics (OB)

Unfortunately, as in Pediatrics, we did not usually see normal deliveries, unless it was a student or the wife of a doctor. We dealt mostly with high-risk pregnancies, which was very difficult for me. And, we often had very small premature babies, which at that time, were difficult to save. In addition, many of them had incurable birth defects. Today, many very tiny babies live and have normal lives.

The Bowel Movement

At that time, new mothers usually stayed in the hospital for several days after delivery. And, some doctors required that the new mother have a bowel movement (BM) before discharge. This was often difficult, because an enema was usually given immediately before delivery.

One woman had many stitches. She confessed to me that she had had a BM in the bathtub, because that was the only way she could do it. She said she cleaned out the bathtub and made me promise not to tell. And I recorded it as a BM, so she could be discharged. I also re-sanitized the tub very carefully!

Accidents

Interns often delivered babies for practice and some of them were a little clumsy. I remember the one who sewed his glove into the episiotomy (stitches) and had to redo it. I also remember one who dropped the new baby into a basin. Fortunately, there were no injuries and I am sure the mothers never knew.

My New Job

When I had a baby several years later in Eitel Hospital, the OB ward was totally full. I was placed in an adjoining Medical Ward.

My roommate was a very elderly lady. This was very weird, but she enjoyed seeing my baby.

After a day or two, I was very bored, but I was required to stay several days until my son could be discharged. (I was a licensed RN by that time.)

I asked if there was anything I could do to help, because the unit was so busy. They said it would be helpful if I charted the vital signs for the unit. So, I was sitting at the nurses' desk in my *bathrobe and paper slippers*, charting. A doctor came up to me and asked, "Who the hell are you?"

The Angry Anesthetist

When I had my baby, I made a deal with the Obstetrician that I would not have anesthesia. We had an overachieving male anesthetist who insisted on giving me morphine and other anesthesia. The female OB doctor made him stop.

While she was finishing after the drug-free delivery, I said to the anesthetist, "If you want to do something helpful, you could go get me a Coke."

This was very insulting to him and he was really angry. However, the doctor made him do it. Later, I received a bill for anesthesia. That was definitely the most expensive Coke I ever had!

Emergency Room (ER)

We had many adventures in the ER. Some were very serious, but some were humorous.

The Vacuum Cleaner

A man came in carrying a canister vacuum cleaner, with the hose still attached to his body. (You can imagine where.) We quickly shuffled him into a private cubicle, where the hose was cut off his penis. (It had created a vacuum and he couldn't get it off.)

We really couldn't understand why the man didn't just cut the hose, rather than bringing the entire vacuum cleaner, but I guess he didn't want to ruin the hose. So, we ruined it for him.

The Potato

Another patient, a very obese lady, came in with complaints of "severe vaginal pain." When she was examined, she had a *very large potato* in her vagina. It had been carefully peeled, with the eyes cut out. She exclaimed, "I can't imagine how it got there. Someone must have put it there when I was asleep." Ouch!

The Soda Bottle

We also had a young woman with a pop bottle in her vagina. A vacuum had been created and she couldn't get it out. We took her to the Dental Clinic to have a hole drilled in the bottle so the vacuum would be released.

The poor young male dental student assigned to the task was so embarrassed. He tried to drill the hole without looking.

Foreign Objects

We always had the proverbial children with the bean in the nose or the ear that you hear about. When a bean is placed in a moist environment, it swells up and becomes difficult to remove. Other children came in with various foreign objects in their bodies. Some had to be removed surgically. I don't remember any serious complications. (There is a story of my son who swallowed many buttons in Chapter 8.)

41

The Messy House

A woman with a permanent tracheostomy (breathing tube in her neck) was choking. Her granddaughter wanted to call the ambulance. The woman's husband would not let the girl call, because he said, "The house is too dirty." By the time the ambulance finally got there, the woman had died.

Ambulance drivers see all types of homes, including "hoarder" situations. They are oblivious to the condition of the home, but are only focused on the victim. In some cases however, the clutter is so bad that rescue people cannot reach the victim or cannot get them out of the house. (Chapter 3)

Mental Health (Psych)

I had many adventures in the Mental Health Unit. This helped me to make the decision to work in Mental Health after retiring from Education. (Chapter 12)

"Keep Him out of the State Hospital"

As a student, I remember caring for a young man about my age. He had a very severe mental illness. They did everything they could to prevent sending him to the state mental hospital, where conditions were very difficult and sometimes archaic, especially for a young person.

In our Psych/Mental Health Ward at the U, we had a padded room and this young man was locked in there most of the time. This was to keep him safe and to prevent him from acting out against others. So, when we wanted to talk to him, we *locked ourselves in with him*. There was one "panic button" on the wall, but if you had an emergency, *you had to get to the button*. I never had any problem with him, however. Sadly, I think he was eventually committed to the state hospital, because there were no other facilities available.

The Sheep

Another man named Murton was from a small town west of Minneapolis. His neighbors called the police. It was reported that he had been having sex with the sheep on his farm. And, the neighbors were concerned. Murton was sent to our hospital for treatment. I don't believe it helped, but he was allowed to return home. (I, the innocent small town girl, had never heard of such a thing.)

The Cribbage Player

We had a well-known dentist as a patient. He was very ill and rarely spoke. However, he loved to play Cribbage. He was amazing, because he could look at his cards and tell you his total points without counting them out like the rest of us, ("15-2, 15-4," and so on.) Other than that, he was mostly unable to care for himself.

The Puzzle Lady

We also had a nonverbal woman who was a master at jigsaw puzzles. She would open the box and lay out the pieces. Then, she would pick up one piece at a time and place it in the puzzle. She never needed to look at the picture. And, she never needed to try a piece to see if it would fit. She could just visualize where each piece should go. It was amazing.

Hot Soup

We had a young man who refused to eat the food served to him.

When we asked why, he said, "It is poisoned." The nurse asked if he would eat if she got him something from the staff cafeteria and he said he thought that would be safe.

So, she came back with a steaming hot bowl of chili. When she took the cover off the steaming chili, he said, "I can't eat that. It's still breathing!"

Therapies

The psychiatric treatments in those days were quire archaic and sometimes barbaric. We had very few medications at that time, so other treatments were used.

For example, they did "regressive shock therapy." This involved giving repeated "shock treatments" (electro-convulsive therapy—ECT) until the person was regressed to childhood. The theory was that if they could regress a person to an age before a traumatic event occurred, they could use psychotherapy to bring the patient back to the current time and they would have erased the traumatic event.

It was very sad to see these regressed adults who were not toilet trained or who could not feed themselves. I also don't think the treatment was very effective. (Regressive shock therapy is no longer used, although controlled ECT is frequently used and is effective in many cases.)

We also did "insulin shock therapy" in the 1950s. The goal was similar to regressive shock. Sometimes, we had to give sugar to a patient, to offset the adverse effects of the extra insulin.

"Hydrotherapy," immersion in water, was also used to calm people.

In some severe cases, a frontal lobotomy (removal of the front part of the brain) was done. These therapies are no longer used today.

Today's treatment relies, in large part, on the use of medications, behavior modification, and talk therapy.

A great deal of therapeutic *Electro Convulsive Therapy* [ECT], previously known as "shock therapy," is also used today.

Some patients are on maintenance ECT, receiving a treatment every two or three weeks. Today, ECT is done in a much more humane way and is very effective in certain cases. (Chapter 12)

Rural Nursing

I went to Glencoe immediately after my wedding for Rural Nursing experience. We stayed in private homes, several students to each home.

It was the middle of winter and extremely cold. We had an old car that would never start (a 1949 Chrysler woodie convertible—I wish I had it today!)

I had to have the battery "jumped" whenever I wanted to start the car to go to Glencoe or to go home. It also used at least a quart of oil for each fifty-five mile trip. I could only make it half-way and then I would need more oil. I could not turn the car off to check or fill the oil or it wouldn't start again. So, I had to convince workers in service stations to put oil in without checking it. (In those days, people did not check their own oil.)

The actual Rural Nursing rotation was almost exactly like my experience at St. Michael's Hospital when I was in High School. And, this experience was helpful later when I was a Public Health Nurse. (Most of today's nursing students do not receive this specific type of experience.)

Public Health Rotation (PH)

For my Public Health experience, I was sent to Alexandria, Minnesota, to work with the School Nurse, Alice, at the high school.

We performed the routine tasks of a school nurse and also made home visits for school concerns. Placement in Alexandria was a special concession to me, because my mother was very ill and I would be able to stay with her (in Sauk Centre) and help her.

I also spent some time with the Director of the Practical Nursing Program there. We had a group class in St. Cloud once a week, to discuss our experiences.

Both of these experiences greatly helped prepare me for positions I held after graduation, since I later did both Public Health nursing (Chapter 3) and School Nursing. (Chapter 4)

I also established a new Practical Nursing Program. (Chapter 7)

TB Rotation at Glen Lake Sanitarium

We had a short rotation at Glen Lake Sanitarium ("the San") working with TB (tuberculosis) patients. This was a special interest of Miss Densford's. A TB rotation in a nursing program was very rare.

One of my classmates contracted TB while on rotation there. She had to spend *almost a year as a patient* in the San. She had to drop out of school and return the next year to graduate.

Later, TB was nearly eradicated in the US as new medications were available, so the San has been repurposed. (Cases of TB have recently emerged in the US, related to immigration of people from various third world countries.)

Many years after my experience at the San, I was required by my employer to have yearly Mantoux (PPD) tests to determine exposure to TB. I am still negative.

My supervisor was amazed, because I had worked in so many places, including the San and Public Health. (In addition, my uncle died of TB, which was pretty much a family secret. In years past, people were very afraid of TB and families didn't want to acknowledge it.)

A very informative book, *The Girl in Building C—The True Story of a Teenage Tuberculosis Patient*, describes a young girl's hospitalization in a sanitarium, her surgeries, and other treatments. She was there for nearly three years, from October, 1943 to September, 1946. (See Bibliography)

The book is dedicated to . . ."the more than fifty thousand people who sought to be healed at one of Minnesota's . . .tuberculosis sanitariums."

Graduation

After graduation from the School of Nursing, I was eligible to take the State Board examination to become a Registered Nurse. I also received a BSN (Bachelor of Science in Nursing) and we were certified as Public Health Nurses.

First, we attended the regular University graduation, with traditional caps and gowns. Then, the Nursing Program had a special capping/graduation ceremony. Here, we received our graduate nursing caps.

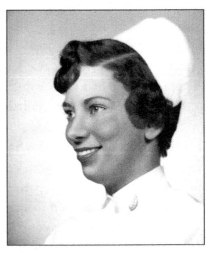

Caroline Rosdahl's graduation photo, showing the Minnesota graduate nursing cap, 1960 (Sisson Studio, Buffalo Minnesota)

The Graduate Nursing Caps

The University's graduate caps were different from our student caps.

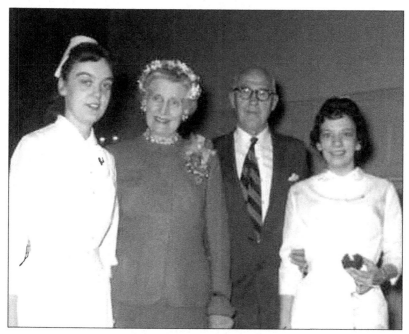

Nursing Graduation, March, 1960—Rosdahl with roommate Judy, Katherine Densford Dreeves, and Mr. Dreeves (BH Media)

Our graduate caps were rounded, with a gathered crown and the "wings" were fastened down. Our caps were patterned after those from the Eastern US and Europe, because the Minnesota program is the oldest continuous university-based program in the U.S. and the first to offer a Bachelor's Degree in Nursing.

We were told that a "little old lady" made the graduate caps, which was most likely true. Of course, I still have my nursing cap. (My husband recently saw an obituary photo in the newspaper and said, "Look at that funny nursing hat." And, I said, "I have one just like it in my office.")

We could tell where a nurse went to school by looking at the cap, since every school's cap was unique. This did cause me a problem later when I worked at Minneapolis General Hospital. (Chapter 5)

Nursing caps went out of favor in about 1975, particularly when more men entered nursing. The caps were a bother sometimes, because they got hung up in the curtains around the bed when you were giving nursing care. But, I was very proud of my cap and hated to give it up. (I understand some uniform shops still sell generic nursing caps, because some people, including nursing assistants, want to wear them.)

SPECIAL STORIES

We had many adventures as nursing students. Some were humorous, but we learned something from all of them.

The Flying Oxygen Tank

During my student rotation working night shift in the Heart Hospital, an orderly dropped an oxygen tank and broke off the top. (Tanks are always supposed to be in a special rack, for safety purposes. However, this orderly was not observing protocol.)

The large, heavy metal "J" tank took off like a jet, flew straight down the long hallway, crashed through a wall and the window, and embedded itself in the lawn outside. This was actually a missile.

Fortunately, no patients were walking around. If anyone had been hit, they would probably have been killed.

My friend and nursing classmate Dee, was also there when this happened. This was an excellent example for us both to use later in our teaching of students. We were able to emphasize the potential danger of gas under pressure. We could point out the importance of always safely securing tanks in a cart or rack.

Fortunately, most hospitals today have a piped-in oxygen supply in each room. But, oxygen tanks are still used in other areas, such as emergency field hospitals, dental offices, nursing homes, clinics, and clients' homes.

The Hopping Senior Citizen

I was working in Urology, where most of the patients were men. Nearly every patient had a leg bag to collect urine. The bag was emptied by removing a plug on the bottom of the bag.

During the night, an elderly gentleman came hopping down the hall on one foot. He was holding the other leg up, so his knee was bent, with that foot off the floor. (If I had tried to do this, I would probably have landed on my face.)

When I asked him what was going on, he said, "I lost my plug!"

Bad Tasting Water

My classmate, Sharon, was caring for an elderly gentleman. She went into his room and he said, "The water in that white pitcher tastes OK, but the water in that silver one really tastes bad." (Of course, the silver thing was his urinal.)

Worms

My classmate, Dee, was caring for a lady named Alicia. She gave the patient an enema and the bedpan was completely filled with the biggest tapeworm anyone in the hospital had ever seen.

The lady was unconcerned and said, "Oh, this is nothing. Everyone where I come from has these worms." The worm was so huge that all the doctors and other nurses came to look at it before the bedpan was dumped.

The Choir at Southdale

We had a nursing student choir. We sang for Christmas at Powell Hall. We also sang for the opening of Southdale, the first enclosed shopping mall in the country. None of us can remember singing anywhere else.

A Sad Powell Hall Story

One Sunday I returned from a weekend at home and was told by my classmates to "lock my door." Since we had no air conditioning, we often left our doors and windows open. Nobody would tell me why I should lock my door. It was a big secret.

I found out some time later that a girl in the dorm had been raped in her bed at knifepoint. They never found out who raped her, but everyone assumed that the man came through the tunnel from the hospital.

Just as an aside. Since it was so hot in our dorm rooms, we sometimes moved our mattresses out onto the roof. This was of course, illegal and dangerous. We had to stop after we got caught.

The Trip to Atlantic City: NSNA Convention

A special highlight of my time at the U was the National Student Nurses' Association (NSNA) convention in Atlantic City, New Jersey, in 1958. I was fortunate enough to win a scholarship to this convention or I would never have been able to go. Several of us from my nursing class went (Nedra Nichols, Sue Doering, Judy Tiede, JoAnn Elliot, and myself).

Two of my childhood girl friends, Dona and Jane, from three-year schools of nursing, also made this trip. (Their photos are in the Introduction to this book.)

We spent three days and two nights on the train to get to Atlantic City. We changed trains in Chicago and somewhere in Pennsylvania, probably Philadelphia.

The last train was a commuter train and I am sure the passengers

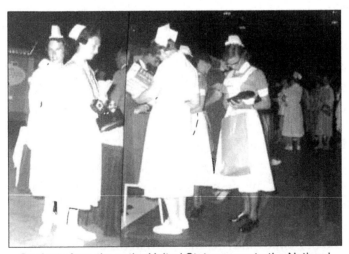

Students from the entire United States came to the National Student Nurses' Association (NSNA) in Atlantic City, New Jersey,1958—each school had a unique student uniform and cap
(CB Rosdahl)

wondered about the group of bedraggled girls who had had no sleep for about two days. We stayed in private homes in Atlantic City.

It was so exciting to see nursing students from all over the country. One day, everyone wore their student uniform and there were many different styles. Some of the girls from the East were wearing black nylons and black shoes with Cuban heels.

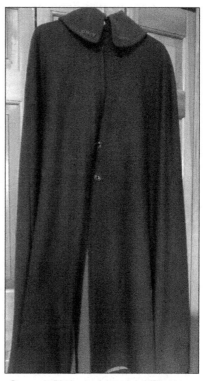

Each school had a distinctive cap and we noticed that many of the Eastern schools had round caps without wings, similar to our graduate caps. Some students had Florence Nightingale-type capes.

It was very interesting to meet students from other areas of the country and to compare notes about their nursing programs. We realized that our program was unique and of the highest quality. We felt very fortunate to be from the University of Minnesota.

Some NSNA students had Florence Nightingale-type nursing capes (CB Rosdahl)

The convention included many interesting and educational meetings, seminars, speeches, demonstrations, and films. We could ask questions and get information and demonstrations about new procedures and products. Advanced education and continuing education opportunities were presented and made available to us as well.

The Drug Salesman

There were displays of many different things, including medical equipment and special procedures. New drugs were displayed and discussed. I met a Parke-Davis salesman and he tried to hustle me. He told me that I could safely go to bed with him, because he had a pill that would prevent me from getting pregnant. I had never heard of such a thing, so I thought he was lying. It turns out his story was true. This was the *beginning of birth control pills*. I did not try them out, however!

The Boardwalk and the Beach

We had some free time and spent it walking the Boardwalk and swimming on the beautiful beach. I had never seen the ocean, so it was a great experience. The entire convention was a wonderful opportunity and I was very grateful that the University gave me the opportunity to go.

Colonel Melody

Some of my classmates were walking on the Boardwalk and they met a distinguished-looking middle-aged gentleman. He knew that we were nursing students attending a national convention. He told them this ridiculous story about being an officer in the Army and working at the Pentagon in Washington D.C. Sure? Right! The girls told him that Judy (Tiede) and I were planning to go to D.C. on our way home. (We were going to visit my Aunt Aldean, Uncle Bob, and Cousin Bobby Dean, who lived in Bethesda, Maryland.)

The girls called us to come meet this man. He said we should call him when we got to D.C. and he would show us around. And, to make the story more ridiculous, he said his name was, of all things, *Colonel Melody*! Really?

He gave us a phone number, hesitating several times to try to remember the number. He said that in order for the switchboard at the Pentagon to put the call through, we would have to give the operator our names, because she screened all his calls.

We knew the whole story was all fiction, trying to impress a bunch of young girls from Minnesota. So we forgot about it and continued our visit in Atlantic City. Our Minnesota friends said "good-bye" and laughingly wished us "good luck in D.C. with Colonel Melody." It was really a big joke.

When we got to Bethesda, Judy and I decided, just for fits and giggles, that we would call the number he gave us and find out what the joke was. We called and an operator said, "U.S. Department of Defense, may I help you?"

This was a shock, but we still thought it was a joke. We gave our names and asked for Colonel Melody. She put us through and a man's voice said, "This is Colonel Phil Melody!"

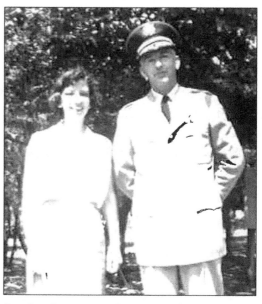

Caroline Bunker and Colonel Philip Buckley Melody, Supervisor of the US Army's Community Relations Program, 1958 (BH Media)

Unbelievably, *the whole story was true* and we later learned that *he supervised the entire Army's worldwide community relations program.* (His rank of Colonel was one step below that of Brigadier General.)

We made arrangements to meet Colonel Melody the next day at Arlington National Cemetery. He invited Cousin Bobby Dean to go sightseeing with us, but my Aunt was so angry, she wouldn't let him go. (When I think about it now, I realize that she couldn't believe we were going off with a total stranger, and an older man at that. I guess she was afraid something bad would happen to us and she would feel responsible . . .and my mother would strangle her.)

However, the next day, we went to Arlington National Cemetery; and it was a very hot day. Colonel Melody showed up in full Army uniform. We had a picnic and then we left with him. My aunt and uncle and Bobby Dean stayed behind . . . and the adventure began.

Colonel Melody's Relationship to Nurses

As the day wore on, Colonel Melody confessed to us that a nurse had, "Saved his life one time." He knew that we were nursing students because he had seen everyone at the NSNA convention.

He did not share any details, but he said that was why he wanted to show us around, "To help pay back the skills and kindness of that nurse and to honor all nurses."

He said, "I just knew you would be good nurses and I am thankful for the patients that you will help in the future." Being nursing students gave us a very unique opportunity that day.

General Maxwell D. Taylor

Colonel Melody showed us all around the Pentagon. He introduced us to many important Army personnel. The most important person we met was General Maxwell D. Taylor, who was *Army Chief of Staff* from 1955 to 1959. Taylor succeeded Matthew B. Ridgeway.

After leaving the Pentagon, General Taylor had a number of other important positions. He was Ambassador to South Vietnam and later, *Chair of the Joint Chiefs of Staff.* He died in 1987 at age eighty-five. (Google Information, 2018)

General Taylor was very pleasant and cordial. Most likely, he rarely had a couple of young girls to visit with. He took us to a theater room and said he was going to show us a very special movie, if we would promise to keep it a secret. He showed us a film of a rocket-type thing and said, "*This is called a satellite. The Army has been secretly developing them. No civilians have ever seen this movie before.* You have to promise not to tell." Not long after that, the first information about satellites was released.

Years later, because I was nurse and an educator, my husband and I were invited to be special guests at a launch of the Space Shuttle in Florida. (Chapter 8)

This certainly reminded me of the trip Judy and I took in 1958. We were so fortunate to have met General Taylor and Colonel Melody and to have seen the movie of one of the first U.S. satellites!

The Washington Monument and Other Special Sites

We stopped at the Washington Monument and it was locked. Colonel Melody called someone and they came and opened it for him! He really was a very important man. Colonel Melody spent the day with us and showed us all the monuments and special places in D.C. He took us to the Officers' Club for a snack. (We were too young to drink.) Of course, we were awed by all of this.

Howard Johnson's

Then Colonel Melody said he was really hot, since he had been wearing his heavy Army uniform all day. He said he would like to stop at his home, which was nearby, so he could change clothes. We had spent every cent we had to buy plane tickets home, because we were going to miss the student train. And of course, we did not have credit cards then.

Colonel Melody left us at the Howard Johnson's Restaurant in Falls Church, Virginia and told us to order dinner for him and ourselves. As we were sitting there, we realized the situation we were in. We got the giggles, because we knew we were completely at his mercy. He could leave us there and we would not be able to pay for three dinners. We had no way to get to the airport and he had all of our luggage in his car.

Of course, Colonel Melody came back and bought us dinner and drove us to the airport. As our plane took off, we could see him standing there watching and waving. He even wrote to us after we got home to make sure we got there safely. And, we corresponded for a couple of years.

Colonel Philip Buckley Melody was one of eight children. He died in 1999 at the age of eighty-nine.

He was a "highly decorated thirty-year career Army Officer, having received, among other decorations, the Bronze Star and the French Croix deGuerre."

He had an MA degree in Education and had graduated from several Army programs.

"He also was one of the few American officers to attend the British

Commando School in Scotland . . . During World War II, Colonel Melody trained underwater demolition assault teams for the invasion of Normandy. When his division liberated Paris, he was chosen to be the *American representative to present Paris back to General De-Gaulle* . . .After D-Day, he assumed command of the 830th Engineer Battalion, which built tactical airfields for the 9th Air Force from Normandy to Berlin . . . After leaving the Army, Melody was Dean of Students at Quinsigamond and Massasoit Community Colleges."(Melody biography: *Geneology.Com*, 2018 and Google, 2018)

A Final Story

Jesus Christ

I was interviewing a new patient on the Medical unit. I asked him his name and he said, "Jesus." (In Spanish, this is pronounced "Hay-soos.")

I didn't exactly know what to say, so I asked if that was his first name. He said it was.

So, I asked him what his last name was and he said, "Christ, you dumb, stupid little kid!"

They didn't teach us how to respond to all situations in nursing school!

CHAPTER 3

PUBLIC HEALTH NURSE

The Job Interview

While I was still a nursing student at the U of Minnesota, I interviewed for the position of Director of the Wright County Public Health Nursing Service (in Buffalo, Minnesota.) I didn't even know where Buffalo was. I had to look it up on a map. (Later, we lived in Buffalo for twenty-five years.)

One reason I was interested in the position was salary. My friends who took positions in "The Cities" were going to be paid about $350 per month. The county job paid $400 per month, plus mileage when I was on the job. (I was already married and we were poor.) Public Health Nursing was included in our nursing curriculum, so in addition to becoming a *Registered Nurse* (RN), I was also eligible for *Certification as a Public Health Nurse* (PHN) at graduation.

To my surprise, I was interviewed in Wright County by a "committee." I was expecting to be interviewed by one or maybe two people. Apparently, committee interviews were a fairly common practice, but I was not expecting it. (Remember, I was a twenty-something student and I had never interviewed for a nursing job before.) We had no preparation in school for obtaining a job. We had no instruction in writing resumes' or interviewing. (Today, much of this information is included in the nursing curriculum.)

When I walked into the room, there were several people there. This group included the County Auditor, Dave Douglas; a member of the County Board of Commissioners, Ruth Homuth; The County Superintendent of Schools, Inez Anderson; the Sheriff, Darrell Wolfe; and the County Probation Officer, Dan Kiernan. I am sure there was also someone from the Welfare Department.

The former nurse had already left, so the position had been vacant for several months. When I think about it now, I imagine they were desperate. They offered me the job, I think on the spot, or maybe the next day. I was living in Minneapolis and planned to commute. I started working in Wright County in approximately January, 1960. I worked weekends and whenever I could during the week.

Waiting for Graduation

I was actually functioning as a *nursing assistant* when I started, since I was not yet licensed. I spent time meeting the other employees of the county, updating myself on the case load and reviewing client charts, making plans for screening programs in the schools, and planning for the reestablishment of the department. I visited some nursing homes and the two hospitals in the county, as well as some of the industries. I also worked on finding volunteers to help with activities, such as immunization clinics.

As soon as I was licensed, I took over the actual duties of the Public Health Nurse. (I was the only Public Health Nurse in Wright County at that time. Now, there are about eighteen PHNs there. Of course, the population of the County has also increased.)

RN Licensure

In those days, nursing graduates took the State Board examination for RN licensure several days or weeks after graduation. Then, the results were mailed out to our homes. (No e-mail.) The test took two days and there were about five sections (including Basic Skills, Med-Surg, Peds, and OB.) Candidates had to pass each section individually. So, the County took a big chance on me, because people often did not pass all the sections on the first try and had to be retested. I could very well not have become licensed immediately.

As an aside, when the results of my State Board exam were mailed to me, I was too nervous to open the envelope. Finally my mother, who was living with me at the time, opened it and told me that I had passed. Now, I was a Registered Nurse and also a Certified Public Health Nurse!

Public Health Nurse Job Responsibilities

I was responsible for fifty-six one-room ungraded "country schools," about twenty town public and parochial schools, about twenty industries, and about twenty nursing homes. Most of these places did not have a licensed nurse on staff. Even the nursing homes did not all have a licensed nurse on duty twenty-four hours a day.

In addition to all these facilities, I had an active public health caseload. It was, of course, an impossible job, but I was too green to know that. So, I plunged in and I really enjoyed the work and the people. And, I REALLY learned a lot. Quickly!

Since I had no actual orientation to the responsibilities of the position, I had to learn as I went along. And, remember, my Public Health rotation was in a high school, so I had really no introduction to home visits, industrial nursing, or nursing homes. I worked for Wright County from January, 1960 to September, 1962. I then was offered a job as a School Nurse and I was excited because I would have summers off. (More about that later.)

General Information

After a short time of commuting fifty miles one-way, from Minneapolis to Buffalo, and getting calls at all hours of the day and night, we decided to move to Buffalo, which was the Wright County seat. My office was in the County Courthouse. (Remember, I had to do a lot of driving during the day also.) Later we built a business in Buffalo (the Dairy Queen), so we stayed there, even though I then was working much closer to Minneapolis.

What Time is It?

We rented an upstairs apartment from Gordon Smith, the manager of the local telephone company. He lived downstairs.

In those days, a live "operator" ran the local town switchboard. ("Number Please.") The night we were moving in, I called the operator to find out what time it was. I didn't have a watch or radio available. We were playing records on the stereo.

When I asked the time, the operator must have thought I was some sort of crank, so she wouldn't tell me what time it was. I called back twice more and tried to explain the situation and she said, "You can just listen to your radio and they will say the time."

I told her I didn't have a radio and she didn't believe me, because she could hear the music. So, she disconnected me again.

Now, I was getting mad, so I called our landlord (Smith) downstairs and explained the situation. I asked him what time it was, because I had to go to work the next day. It was something like 1:30 AM. Smith was really angry with the operator.

Apparently, after that they put a red light on our number at the switchboard (like the firemen had.) So after that, whenever I picked up the phone, I got instant service.

On Call 24/7

People began to call me whenever they had a question or a medical concern (so I was actually doing triage.) Many times, I had to tell them to call the ambulance or go to their doctor. Occasionally, I would go to the home to see if I could help. (People even called me with questions about their sick pets!)

Since I lived in a small town, everyone knew me and usually knew where I was at any given time. (Population: about 3000.) For example, one night, there was a Courthouse Christmas party and someone called me.

The operator said, "Oh, I know she isn't home tonight. I'm sure she's at the party." So, she put the call through to the party (and I was there.) There was very little privacy.

The Facilities in the County

There were a number of facilities that I visited during my tenure as the County Nurse. None of them had a full-time nurse, and most relied totally on the County Nurse for healthcare services.

Nursing Homes

The nursing homes were the worst part of my job. Most of them didn't have an RN or LPN on duty at night. Maybe, they had to have one during the day, or once a week, or on call. I never was able to figure out the regulations (which were very few.) In any event, most of the conditions were deplorable. When you walked in the door, you immediately had to adjust to the odor, mostly of urine.

On my first visit to a nursing home, I almost turned around and walked out. It seemed hopeless. In most of the nursing homes, it appeared that the residents were in bed most or all of the day. Some were up in wheelchairs. It seemed that none of them were able to walk or were assisted to try. The residents all looked neglected.

Most of the residents had no idea what was going on, because there were no activities, no information about current events, or rehabilitation. Most of the nursing homes did not even have a TV. Some of the clients were totally confined to their rooms. Very few of the residents had any visitors; their families had abandoned them.

I had no idea where to start. I tried to get the owners of the facilities to improve the conditions, but I am not sure it did much good.

Since then, Minnesota has passed strict laws regulating these facilities and today the conditions are much, much better. Unfortunately, I was unable to spend much time in the nursing homes, because of the extent of my job. I regret that, but I don't know if I could have done anything at that time to improve the situation.

Holding Hands

One day, I went to one of the nursing homes and an elderly couple was sitting in the lounge holding hands. I commented to the staff that it was nice that they could be together. However, the staff person said, "It would be nicer if they were married to each other, rather than to other people."

Industries

There were several fairly large industries in the county, including canning factories, which were quite dangerous. I visited the industries and tried to make suggestions to improve safety for their workers. (We did have a couple of accidents, but no deaths while I was there.)

I encouraged the industries to install eyewash stations, First Aid kits, and fire extinguishers. I tried to have a person in each industry designated as the Safety Person. They taught people how to use the eyewash stations and fire extinguishers, monitored the number of accidents, rewarded employees for accident-free periods of time, and showed First Aid films.

I tried to train the Safety people in simple First Aid techniques, including when to call an ambulance. These people worked hard to maintain safe environments and the accident rate in the industries was lowered while I was in the County.

Each industry had a physician assigned as their resource person. None of these industries had a nurse on staff. The industry safety volunteers were very helpful. Today, regulations are much stricter and it is safer to work in an industry such as a canning factory or manufacturing plant.

Rural Schools

Imagine being responsible for basic screening and referral for all the students in fifty-six one-room rural schools, spread all over the county! Inez Anderson was the County Superintendent, supervising all these schools. Most schools had eight to fifteen students, either from first to eighth grade or ending at sixth grade. Students then were old enough to either quit school or transfer to a larger town school.

In these rural schools, one teacher had to teach all the subjects for all the grades. There were advantages and disadvantages of this type of education. Younger students could listen to the older students' classes and learn from that. And, the older students often helped the younger students, gaining valuable experience. (Many students were in classes with their brothers and sisters.)

The only problem could be that if the teacher was not doing a good job, the students had *her* (almost always a woman) for their entire grade school years. However, most of the rural teachers were wonderful. They did an amazing job, probably akin to some of today's home schooling. I can't imagine how difficult it was, but they did it.

I made sure to *visit each rural school at least once a year*. On these visits, I did basic vision and hearing screening, as well as consultation regarding specific health conditions. Occasionally, I was asked to do a scoliosis or other health screening. I referred any pertinent cases to the children's parents, to manage follow-up care. In more difficult cases, I made a home visit to discuss the problem with the parents. In rare cases, I needed to take a student to the doctor, because the parents were unable to do so. (I would imagine that today the nurse is not permitted to transport a student, for legal reasons.) In some schools, teachers requested that I do a basic "sex education" class for the students. Now, this is a major challenge if some of the students are five or six years old and both boys and girls are in one room!

In the rural schools, students brought a sandwich or something for lunch. Sometimes, the teacher prepared a big pot of soup or stew to supplement the bag lunch. This was often kept on the pot-bellied stove in the middle of the room, which also heated the schoolroom. The teacher, of course, had to come early to light the stove in the morning. She also rang the bell, to call the children to school.

Most of these schools did not have running water or may have had a pump only for drinking water. They often used an outhouse as a bathroom, which was VERY cold in the winter.

Some of these schools did not have electricity until the REA (Rural Electrification Association) went through, sometimes as late as the 1950s or '60s. The children usually walked to school. (Riding a bike was difficult on the gravel roads.) In some cases, if they lived further away, they rode their horses and tied them out behind the school to graze for the day.

1967 legislation in Minnesota did away with these rural schools and they were all closed by about 1969. Some were converted to homes or town halls; some were abandoned.

A Stolen Lunch
One little boy came to school frequently without a lunch. When the teacher asked about this, he said, "That big black dog is always waiting in the ditch for me to walk by and he grabs my lunch." When this was investigated, the child's story was true. So, guess who had to go over and talk to the owner of the dog? (There are many facets to Public Health Nursing.)

The Kidnapped Teacher
One day, I went to visit a small rural school. I called out and everyone was gone. Then, I heard a faint cry of "**Help!**" I went around to the back and the teacher was *securely tied to a tree*. (Remember: in those days, a person could teach in a rural school after two years of college, regardless of what classes were taken.)

The young teacher in this school was new to teaching; it was early

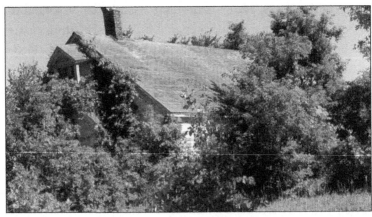

Abandoned Country Schoolhouse (U.S. Highway 12, west of Delano, Minnesota)—these schools were abolished in the late 1960s
(CB Rosdahl)

in her first year. She was probably only nineteen or twenty years old. Some of the boys were almost as old as she was and were certainly bigger.

In addition to tying her to the tree, the boys had also laid a fire at her feet. (Fortunately, they did not light it.) I can't imagine what would have happened if I had not come that day. We *never did see that teacher again* — she apparently quickly found another occupation. ☺

The teachers, both rural and in town, often rented a room in a neighborhood home. This could be uncomfortable, because usually they were living with some of their students. (My family usually had a teacher renting a room from us when I was young.)

Town Schools

The vision, hearing, and basic health screening duties in the larger public and parochial schools were the same as those in the rural schools. However, there were many more students in these schools, and since some of them were high schools, many of the students were older. I organized a group of volunteers to assist with this task. The volunteers were very helpful with set-up and recording for these screenings.

More home visits were needed for the town school students, simply because there were so many more students. In addition, it was my responsibility to make sure that students in athletics had a valid physical exam before participating. Sometimes, follow-up with parents was necessary, as a result of these physicals. Some students had never seen a doctor or dentist and had never had immunizations. This was also discussed with the parents.

I was also responsible for teaching sex education in many of these schools. The boys and girls were taught separately. (Many times, only the girls received this education.) Most of the teachers were too embarrassed to teach these classes, so I was on my own. And, remember, I was only about fiver years older than some of the students.

The Deaf Child

During one of my school visits, I was told that Tommy who was four-years-old, would not be coming to school, because he had never learned to talk. When I tested him, I discovered he was totally deaf. I had a conference with Tommy and his parents and he was referred to a hearing specialist. After he got appropriate hearing aids, he quickly learned to talk and did well in school.

Edwin and Leland

One town school had two students who were severely mentally challenged. They were simply placed in the back of a classroom and given coloring books or something else to keep them busy. They were passed on from grade to grade without taking part in any of the classes. (At that time, there were no facilities for special education.)

We had to bring in bigger desks for these two boys when they were in the lower grades, because they were older and larger than other students in the class. They just remained until they were old enough to quit school.

It was very sad, because today they would have been given special classes and probably would have been able to work in a sheltered workshop and learn to care for themselves. I referred them to the Welfare Department, but appropriate training facilities were not available in their area.

I learned many years later that one of them (Edwin) had become a farmer and was doing well.

SPECIAL STORIES

I had many adventures as the County Nurse. Some were humorous and some were challenging.

The Speeding Ticket

One evening, I was supposed to speak at Howard Lake High School. (I have no idea what the topic was.) I was driving from Buffalo and I was late. I came to the stop sign on County Highway 25, entering US Highway 12, and there was a car coming from my left. So, I sped up a little to get in front of him.

He was following me very closely; the faster I went, the faster he went. This made me nervous, so I sped up even more. When I was going about eighty miles an hour, the *Highway Patrol* turned on his red lights and siren and pulled me over.

I knew I had to talk fast to explain and avoid a ticket, if possible, so I started talking as soon as he approached my car. I said, "I know I was going too fast, but you scared me." After letting me talk for a while about speeding, he said, "I wasn't going to give you a ticket for speeding. I was going to give you a ticket for running the stop sign!"

I told him I was the County Nurse and I was supposed to give a speech and I was late. I of course, looked very young (I *was very young*) and he obviously did not believe me. "So, you're the County Nurse, huh? Well, I'll just give you an escort and then you'll get there faster."

So, he followed me right into the door of the school and did not leave until the moderator said, "Oh good, here's Mrs. Rosdahl now." I walked up onto the stage and the officer left. If I had been lying, I would have gotten a ticket for sure.

The Child with Cerebral Palsy

I went on a home visit one day and found a child of about twelve lying stomach-down on a mechanic's creeper. (The scooter used by mechanics to repair the bottoms of cars.) When I asked about this, I was told that the child had cerebral palsy and the creeper was the only way he could get around. It was very unfortunate and I was sure something could be done to help him. At that time, there was almost no assistance for these cases.

The boy had never been to school, because there were no facilities for children with disabilities. Of course, there were no computers, so distance learning was not an option. I contacted the local Shriners' lodge and the boy was taken to their hospital in the Twin Cities for evaluation. His parents could not afford special care or equipment, so the Shriners furnished him with a battery-operated wheelchair and trained him how to use it.

Special transportation was arranged and the child was then able to go to school. We also arranged for him to have an individual tutor to help him catch up with his peers. I can't imagine missing so many years of school, but he studied hard and did well. He eventually graduated from high school at the age of twenty-one. I was very proud of him and I hope he did well in his future life.

Trips with the Sheriff
If the Sheriff suspected that someone was badly hurt *or dead*, he usually asked me to accompany him to the scene, because he didn't want to go alone.

The Root Cellar
One day in mid-winter, a report came in that an elderly couple had not been seen for several days. So, we were called to do a "welfare check." The couple lived on a farm in the country and it was bitterly cold. We were afraid we would find them dead. When we got there, we banged on the door and there was no answer. The Sheriff finally broke into the house. We discovered that there was a root cellar under the kitchen floor.

When we went in, the couple had been living in the root cellar for several days, because they had run out of fuel oil. They had built a small wood fire there (it's a wonder they didn't suffocate) to keep warm. They had several dogs in the root cellar with them. They were all subsisting on sweet potatoes (dogs and people.)

The husband had active TB (tuberculosis) and was very thin and sick looking. The wife was very heavy and seemed to be doing fine. We then contacted the Welfare Department and suitable medical care was located for the husband. He spent some time in the TB sanitarium, but he recovered.

The Flood
The Crow River floods almost every spring. One year, it was particularly high and Delano, Minnesota was seriously affected. First, the Sheriff and I went around in a boat, rescuing people off their roofs and out of trees. A couple of people were trapped in flooded cars.

Later, we had to organize an immunization clinic to prevent typhoid, dysentery, and other diseases, because the city water had been contaminated. Since that time, a dike has been constructed to help prevent flooding in the city. But, many buildings near the river have also been removed.

Auto Accidents

Many times, if there was a bad auto accident, I would be asked to go to the scene and help. (I drove a very unique *pink and black and white Dodge* that had belonged to my parents, so everyone in the county knew the car.) If I drove past an accident, the Sheriff would flag me down to stop and help.

The "ambulance" in Buffalo was also used as the town hearse, so you could not stand up. The vehicle was like a station wagon, the same type used in Sauk Centre when I was a Nursing Assistant. You had to kneel to assist a victim.

The ambulance drivers had NO medical training of any kind. All they wanted to do was load up the victim and drive to the nearest hospital or doctor's office. Sometimes, I had to fight with the drivers to let me stabilize the victim a little before loading the person into the ambulance. This was similar to my later experiences at Minneapolis General Hospital. (Chapter 5)

Obviously, procedures have changed greatly since that time. Today's ambulances are true rescue vehicles, with highly trained personnel and the latest medical and rescue equipment. Victims are stabilized before transport and the Paramedics can stand up and move around in the vehicles.

Changing a Tire

One day while I was working for the County, I had a flat tire and was stopped on the shoulder of the road preparing to put on the spare. Two young men in Army uniforms stopped and said they would help me.

Unfortunately, neither of them had a clue as to how to do it. They fumbled around and got the tire changed, with my instructions. But, I was terrified they would drop my car on the road in the process. Their hearts were in the right place though, and the tire got changed.

Immunization Clinics

In addition to basic health screening, we planned immunization clinics, available to all rural and town schools at least once a year. I had a number of local volunteers who helped. We did eight to ten clinics throughout the County, so students from all the schools would have the opportunity to attend.

We gave basic immunizations at these clinics and nearly all the students took advantage of the opportunity. (I think the charge was about $1.00 and if a child could not afford it, the immunizations were free.) We also had clinics for TB (Mantoux, PPD) testing. For all the clinics, a volunteer physician gave the actual injections, but local citizen volunteers helped me set everything up.

I remember situations when the older boys, football players, would pass out while watching people get injections. The little children were mostly unconcerned.

After a Mantoux testing clinic, I had to return two days later to assess the results. If anyone tested Positive, they were referred to their physician. I then had to follow up to make sure they saw their doctor. I also had to follow up to make sure any ordered treatment was obtained. I often needed to meet with parents to discuss these procedures.

I remember one doctor (Dr. G.) who would come to do immunizations in his tiny sports convertible. He had to drive with the top down, so there was room for his golf clubs to stick out in the back seat. Wonder where he went after the clinic was over? ☺

Today, immunizations and PPD tests are often given by nurses or pharmacists, as well as physicians.

Reusing Needles and Syringes

We *reused syringes and needles*, sterilizing them between clinics. We took the glass syringes apart, rinsed them out, and spread them on a towel-covered tray. The needles were all checked for burrs and *any jagged spots were burnished out* before they were reused. These materials were all taken to the Buffalo Hospital to be autoclaved (sterilized). (Mrs. Feckler, the Director of Nursing, was my buddy. She probably felt sorry for me and was willing to help out.)

We never had any problems or infections as a result of reusing needles and syringes. Today's nurses would collapse if they knew how we did it in the "olden days!"

Once in Waubun!

One day about four of us Public Health nurses were traveling around in rural Northern Minnesota, doing Mantoux (PPD) clinics. Each student had to fill out a form printed on a card the size of a small recipe card. This card requested the student's vital information. It included name, address, phone number, sex, parents' names, doctor's name, allergies, and any pertinent health history.

One young girl had written in the very small space for sex, "Once in Waubun." (Waubun is a tiny town in Northern Minnesota.) We decided among ourselves that it was a good thing it was only once, because that space on the card was very small. We suggested to her that she put an " F " in that spot, for female. But, "Once in Waubun" became the battle cry of our group.

Administration

Department of Health Supervision

The State Department of Health decided, since I was a new Public Health Nurse, I needed supervision. They sent a woman named Joan S to "supervise" me. She insisted on spending a half day each week with me. She wanted to "check my charting" and discuss my cases. It didn't seem like she had any actual Public Health Nursing experience. I didn't feel she helped me at all and it took away from the time I desperately needed for my work. I think she was trying to justify her own position. Her visits to me continued for about a year.

Wonderful Secretary

When I started, the County furnished me with a secretary, Lois Mueller. She was young, but very capable. She had been there for a while before I came, so she knew the lay of the land. She was very nice and we became good friends. (She continued to work for the County in the Welfare Department for about twenty five years after I left.)

"Charting" on Tape

While I was working at the County, I was still a friend with the guys in Industrial Education at the U. Here, my time hanging out with them in the "Shack" paid off. (Chapter 6) They helped me invent a means to do charting without having to sit and write evening out. (The nurses previously had returned to the office every day to do their charting after making their home visits. This took away from the time they could spend seeing clients. I felt this was a waste of time.)

Lois was in the office all day and had time to type out my notes. So, the guys designed a converter for me, which enabled me to plug a reel-to-reel tape recorder into the cigarette lighter of my car. Sometimes, I would go over a bump and the recorder would miss a few beats. If I had to slam on the brakes, I had to grab the recorder so it wouldn't slide off the seat. Sometimes, I would play a song on the radio for Lois.

But, Lois could type my notes and I was able to make more home visits. And I didn't waste all the time while I was driving. I should have patented the invention. Maybe I could be a millionaire now. ☺

About forty years later, my good friend, Marj Provo, worked for Wright County. She had some of the same clients I had had and my charting was still there.

Cast of Characters

Marion

There were several very interesting people working with me at the County. My best buddy was Marion, a Social Worker. She was very funny. We often made home visits together, especially to Myrtle C.

Robert

Robert P. also worked for the County. When he and his wife had a son, they called him "the Boy." Then, they had a daughter and she was called "the Girl." Their third child was called "the Baby." We all thought it was good they never had any more children, because they had run out of names! (We never knew the children's real names.)

Dan Kiernan

Dan, the County Probation Officer, was very funny and was always joking around and playing jokes on people. He drove a small Volkswagen bug. One night a bunch of us were at his home. We went out to the garage and turned his car around so it was crosswise in the single-car garage. It barely fit. The next morning Dan was very late to work, because he had to go back and forth an inch at a time to get his car out of the garage.

You could always count on Dan and the Social Workers to assist in a difficult situation, but we did enjoy finding a joke we could play on Dan.

Dave Douglas

Dave was the County Auditor. He was quite serious and was a number of years older than the rest of us. The significant thing about Dave is that his son, Bruce, worked for us at our Dairy Queen. Bruce was a really good kid. He and I took Dilly Bars to the County Fair and did lots of other things for the DQ. He later became an attorney in Buffalo.

A Special Story

One of the county workers had been widowed very young and never had any children. Later, she was traveling in Europe and met a man, Talai Abbar, on the train. He was from one of the United Arab Emirates and he wooed her relentlessly. (She later learned that having an American wife was a status symbol in his country, particularly if the wife was overweight. Then, people would believe that the man was wealthy.)

She and Talai were married and lived for a while in her hometown in Minnesota. Now her name was Madame Talai Abbar. Things were going well, but Talai continually begged her to come to his home country to meet his family. She had misgivings, but finally she relented and went.

Once she got to Abbar's country, she was basically a captive. She had to dress in the traditional manner. "The traditional dress . . . is the *abaya*, a thin, flowing cloak that covers the [entire] body," so only the feet, hands and face are showing. The arms are totally covered. (In some cases, the face is covered, so only the eyes are showing.) Other clothing is worn under the abaya. The head is covered by the *hijab*, which covers the entire head. (Google information, 2019)

As a woman, she had no rights and was not allowed to drive, to go anywhere unaccompanied, or to leave. Alcohol was not permitted. She finally escaped with the assistance of the U.S. Embassy and returned to Minnesota. (The film, "Not Without my Daughter" describes a similar situation.)

Favorite Clients

Nutmeg

Nutmeg was a chubby middle-aged lady who kept getting pregnant or getting VD/STIs (sexually-transmitted infections). Marion, the Social Worker, and I tried to decide how we might break this cycle. (Remember, there was almost no birth control available in those days.) We talked to Nutmeg about the situation and she said, "Maybe if you could write me a letter . . ."

So, we wrote a letter on county letterhead and gave it to Nutmeg. The letter said something to the effect of, "Nutmeg cannot go to bed with you, because we said so." And, both Marion and I signed it. Nutmeg kept the letter in her very dirty, greasy bra. Apparently, she pulled it out and showed it to gentlemen when needed.

Whenever we saw Nutmeg, we asked her to show us the letter. When it became so filthy it was unreadable, we wrote her a new one.

But, it worked. Nutmeg kept from getting pregnant and she did not contract any more STIs.

Nurses have to do whatever works and sometimes this takes imagination!

MaryAnn

MaryAnn was a little old single lady living on a farm with her two unmarried brothers. She had a large wound on her leg and that's why I was asked to visit her. Each time I drove into the driveway, the barrel of a shotgun would come out the window. When they saw it was me, they would lock up the "killer dogs" and invite me in. (It's important to remember; I was too dumb to be scared. I trusted everyone. And, I never had any trouble.)

It is hard to describe MaryAnn's house. The windows were so coated with grease and dirt, you could barely see outside. There was junk all over. Today, we would refer to her as a "hoarder." (Remember, I am from a small town middle-class family, with a very neat and tidy Norwegian mother. I really did not know people lived like this.)

MaryAnn wore bib overalls, some sort of t-shirt, long wool socks, and four-buckle overshoes. All the time. Even in bed. Her bed was in the "living room" and it consisted of a bare mattress (with stripes), an uncovered pillow (with stripes), and a blanket or two. No sheets or pillowcases. When I came, she would throw back the blanket and get out of bed, overshoes and all.

Her leg wound looked terrible. But, she said, "I put goose grease on it and it's getting better." The long wool socks mostly covered the wound. She never changed them, but when her toes went through the ends of the socks, she would just roll them up at the toe. When the socks got too short, she got a new pair. I don't know if she ever changed her other clothes.

The three siblings ate at a table in the main room. They each had their own plate, so they "didn't have to wash dishes." There were other dishes and things on the table. And their huge orange tabby cat was usually stretched out on the table among the clutter. He helped clean the plates, I am sure.

One day, I went there and saw *huge eggshells* on the table. Not being a farm girl, I had no idea what they were. When I asked, MaryAnn said, "Those are goose eggs. And, there's the goose." And, sure enough, the goose was walking around in the house.

Another day I went there and MaryAnn asked if I would like something to eat. "We just ate and there's some left." MaryAnn indicated a large bowl of something white, with a spoon sticking out. I declined, saying I had just eaten. (I knew I would probably die if I ate there, because I hadn't built up resistance to their microorganisms.) Then, MaryAnn picked up the spoon and the entire coagulated contents of the large bowl came out with it. Good thing I wasn't hungry!

MaryAnn was a good soul and her wound eventually healed. She continued to use the goose grease, along with some medication prescribed for her, which I brought with me each visit, so she wouldn't lose it.

Two Large Families

I had two large families to visit. Both lived in the country and both were poor. *But, the contrast between the two was striking.*

One woman had eight children, with the oldest being about ten-years-old. She gave total care to her mother who had suffered a stroke and was mostly bedridden. Her house was a complete shambles, with trash and litter everywhere. But, her mother's bed and her mother were spotless. They were very clean and well cared for. Mother was well fed, her hair was always fixed, and she seemed happy. The daughter made sure Mother did her prescribed exercises every day and read to her. However, caring for Mother was the only thing this very busy mother had time for. So, the rest of the home was a mess.

The other family had about the same number of children. But, in this family, the mother was very organized. Each child had a special job. This house was very old, but neat and clean. I remember that the job of the two-year-old little boy was to wash the wooden stairs every day with a pail of soapy water and a scrub brush. And, he was very proud of this accomplishment. All the other children had jobs appropriate to their ages.

Both families were happy and enjoyed each other's company. But, the contrast between the conditions of the two homes was striking.

Myrtle C

One could write an entire book about Myrtle. She lived a few miles from my office and was a major character. She and her husband were both severely mentally challenged, in addition to chronic mental illness.

However, Myrtle was very good-hearted. They had seven or eight children, half of whom were of normal intelligence. They were usually placed in foster care as children, because Myrtle was unable to care for them. (One daughter was intelligent and very pretty. One year, she was part of her High School Homecoming court.)

Myrtle's house was of course, a complete disaster. She had a traditional kitchen set, the kind with padded plastic seats and chrome legs. However, all the seats and seat backs were gone, so if you wanted to sit down, you balanced a board on top of the chrome legs to sit on.

The house was so dirty that Marion the Social Worker and I wore raincoats when we went there, so we dared to sit down. "Oh, Myrtle, it might rain today." A raincoat was also used if we had to transport Myrtle somewhere. In that case, Myrtle would be asked to wear a special raincoat kept inside out in the trunk of my car.

"Daddy" and the Laundry

One day, I asked how Myrtle's husband "Daddy" was doing at the State Mental Hospital. "Oh," she said, "He's having an awful time." It seemed he had been assigned to work in the laundry. "He just can't make all those decisions." He had been assigned to separate the clothes that were *white from those that were not white*. And, it was too difficult for him. He finally was taken out of the laundry. Occasionally, he came home for a few days.

"Daddy" and Myrtle's Brother

Myrtle's brother sometimes visited their house; Daddy did not like the brother. There were open heat registers between the first and second floors. Daddy would stand over the upstairs register and when the brother walked below him, Daddy would pee on the brother's head.

Peeling Potatoes and Storing Meat

One day, I went to Myrtle's house and she was standing near the stove, with a huge pot of water boiling. She had fresh potatoes out of someone's garden, so there were clumps of dirt on them. She was peeling them and dropping the *peelings, the eyes, and the dirt* into the pot with the peeled potatoes.

When I asked about this, she answered, "Marion said I should peel potatoes before I cook them." (What Marion neglected to tell Myrtle was that only the peeled potatoes should go into the water and not the dirt and the peelings.)

Once, their refrigerator broke down, so they had meat hanging all over the house. But, worse than that was when their toilet stopped working, because then they used the bathtub!

"Fixing" The Washing Machine

One day, Myrtle called me all in a panic. "You gotta' come right away! My blankety-blank kid broke my washing machine." I told Myrtle I didn't know how to fix washing machines. But, she was hysterical. "It's an emergency!"

I could hear the child screaming in the background, so I decided I had better drive over and see what was going on. The washing machine was plugged in near the ceiling into a combination socket for a light bulb and a cluster plug. The young boy, about three years old, was in the washing machine, up to his chest in soapy water.

One tennis-shoed foot was wedged under the agitator, which was still trying to move back and forth, making the tennis shoe squeak loudly. (Now, all she had to do was pull the plug, stopping the machine, but she didn't think of that.)

I unplugged the machine, removed the agitator, and got the kid out. So—I guess I *do know how to fix a washing machine,* even though this was not included in my nursing education!

Myrtle wouldn't tell me how the kid got into the machine. However, I firmly believe that she decided to *wash him and his clothes at the same time*. He was so little; he couldn't have gotten into the machine by himself. We were lucky he didn't drown. Myrtle promised to be more careful with the washing machine in the future. And, I didn't add "washing machine repair" to my nursing resume'.

MISCELLANEOUS STORIES FROM THE "NAKED CITY"

There are so many stories from my time as a Public Health Nurse it is difficult to decide which ones to include. Following are a few samples.

New Mother Visits

I made at least one visit to most new mothers. This was interesting, because I didn't have any children and had really never taken care of tiny babies. All I had to go on was my nursing education. So, mostly we learned together. I hope I helped at least some of them. I tried to answer their questions and give them support. I could provide them with brochures giving advice for new mothers. And, occasionally, the local hospital had a new mother class that I could recommend to them.

Killer Geese

I frequently went to a remote farm in the northern part of the county. These people had a small flock of geese. It is possible that they were trained to kill intruders. However, I have heard that geese are just naturally territorial and will attack people they don't know.

When I drove into their yard, the geese would meet my car, squawking, flapping their wings, and pecking at my car. If the people wanted to see me, they would lock up the geese. If they didn't want to see me, they would just let the geese carry on and I would give up and leave. I never dared to get out of the car when the geese were outside.

The Cat on the Clothesline

An elderly lady, (probably about the age I am now) had a cat she dearly loved. She was afraid the cat would run away. (Now, you and I know that if you feed a cat, he/she is usually yours forever.)

Anyway, she liked to let the cat get fresh air, so she would hook him to a chain on her wire clothesline. The only problem was that the chain was so heavy the cat couldn't sit up straight, let alone move. But, the cat got fresh air!

I was worried that a neighborhood dog would bother the cat, so I got the woman to promise to sit outside and watch when the cat was tied up. So, the cat was safe and the woman also got fresh air.

Moving On

I left the county to become the School Nurse at Hopkins High School. I had enjoyed my two-and-a-half-plus years as the County Nurse and I really learned a lot. It was also a vivid awakening to be exposed to the real "Naked City." I did not know people lived like that. I learned to communicate with people from all walks of life and of all ages. Mostly, I learned that people all have different life styles and these are not necessarily all bad or all good. And people are mostly good, no matter what kind of living conditions they may have. Everyone tries his or her best.

It was a great first job. And, a unique orientation to the whole wide world of nursing in the Naked City!

CHAPTER 4

SCHOOL NURSE

By virtue of my nursing degree from the U, I was also eligible to become a Certified School Nurse. In 1962, I decided that school nursing would be better than being the County Nurse. For one thing, I would get summers off. However, that didn't work out, because we could not afford for me to be off in the summer. So I had to work somewhere else during summers. (Minneapolis General Hospital—Chapter 5)

The Mound Interview
We lived in Buffalo, Minnesota, and there was a School Nurse position in Mound, which was fairly close. I had never been to Mound. (Little did I know that I would later live in Mound for twenty-five years!) So I applied, and at the interview, the Superintendent said, "You understand you will have to move to Mound in order for us to hire you." I told him I lived in Buffalo and we owned a business there (Buffalo Dairy Queen), so I could not move.

That was the end of the interview. However, interestingly, the person they hired also lived in Buffalo. She rented a room in Mound, so she had a fake Mound address. But, she continued to live in Buffalo. It was interesting that she misrepresented her address to get the job. I don't think she worked in Mound very long. I don't know if they ever discovered she really lived in Buffalo.

The Hopkins Interview

Next, I interviewed for a School Nurse position in the Hopkins School District. The Superintendent, Mr. Tanglen, said the same thing—"You will have to live in Hopkins. All of our staff people are required to live in the District."

I told him I could not move and then after talking to me for a while, he said, "Okay, we will hire you, but if you are ever unable to get here because of the weather, you will have to move to Hopkins." So, I drove thirty-three miles one-way through blizzards and floods (in my Volkswagen bug), but I always got there. Other staff and teachers, who lived in Hopkins, only a few blocks away, sometimes could not get out of their driveways and could not get there, but I always made it. I worked at Hopkins from Fall, 1962 through Spring, 1966 (four school years).

L. H. Tanglen was Superintendent of Schools in Hopkins for twenty-two years until his retirement in 1966. An elementary school is named after him. When he started in 1944, the enrollment was 950 students.

He engineered the consolidation of seven school districts into one. When he retired, the enrollment had grown to more than 9,500. "*Mr. Tanglen believed the combining of all resources into one unified district made it possible to upgrade our school system second to none.*" (Hopkins Historical Society, 2002)

The Bug

My old Volkswagen (VW) bug was difficult/impossible to start in the winter. I either had to build a charcoal fire under it (in an oil drain pan) or carry the battery inside. So in the winter, when I got to school, I carried the heavy battery into my office for the day and then carried it back out, in order to go home.

Then when I got home, because we didn't have a garage, I carried the battery back into the house for the night and back out in the morning. I got pretty good at installing batteries! The VW had almost no heater or defroster, so in the winter I had to shift and steer the car with one hand and scrape ice with the other hand all the way to school, so I could see to drive.

Then, the engine went out of the VW. It was very difficult to find anyone to repair the car, because *most mechanics did not have metric wrenches at that time.* I finally located a man from Germany who could fix it. I had him order a new engine and when it arrived, all the instructions were in German. Fortunately, the mechanic spoke German.

As soon as the new engine was installed, I traded the VW for a Chevy. The Chevy was the first car I had ever had that had seat belts. These seat belts later saved my life and the life of my child. (Chapter 5)

School Nurse Adventures

I was assigned to be at Hopkins High School three days a week and Alice Smith Elementary School two days a week. They really didn't want me to make home visits, because they wanted me to be at school at all times, in case of emergency. My secretary, Marge Holm, was a three-year RN, so she was at the High School to do first aid when I wasn't there. I had many adventures in Hopkins.

Alice Smith Elementary School

The principal, Mrs. Harrison, was not married, although apparently she must have been married at some point. (She married again later in life.) She wanted to be in charge of everyone and was demanding. I think some people liked her, but certainly not everybody. She was really frustrated that I was not at her school full-time and didn't report directly to her.

One day, the "real" Alice Smith came to visit the school. She was older, but very sharp. I was very honored to meet the person for whom the school was named.

I had many of the same duties at Alice Smith as I had performed when I was the County Nurse, including vision and hearing screening, immunization clinics, and sex education classes. Occasionally, I was allowed to make a home visit. I did more scoliosis screening and teaching there than I had done before. (Mrs. Harrison was embarrassed about the sex education classes and never came to that session.)

The Exhausted Student

One day a girl of about ten was referred to me by her teacher. I was told that this young girl was always very tired and fell asleep in class. When I talked to the girl, she told me, "It is hard to sleep, because my mother has so many 'uncles' that come to visit at night. Then, I have to sleep on the couch or the floor." (Of course, Mom had a little business going.) We talked to the mother and she made changes in her life so the child could get more sleep. (Sometimes, the girl had to stay with her grandmother.)

The "Head of Household" Bonus

Hopkins paid a bonus of $250 to a person who was head of household. This apparently meant, "Only if you were a man." One of the teachers at Alice Smith was an unmarried lady who was totally responsible for the financial support and care of her elderly parents. She petitioned for the bonus, but it was *denied because she was a woman*. Part of the sexual discrimination we have all lived through for many years!

The Pastor

Another Alice Smith teacher left teaching to become a Lutheran Pastor. She served at Mount Olivet Church in Minneapolis for a number of years. She was married to a man named "Butch." I had known him through my roommate, Judy. Both Judy and Butch were very active at YMCA camp Widjiwagan in the Boundary Waters Wilderness Canoe Area. It's truly a small world.

Hopkins High School

I had many adventures at the high school. Students would stop in my office just to talk. Some of them faked illness just so they could come to the nursing office. They talked to me about many problems—sex, birth control, pregnancy, girl friends, boyfriends, or problems at home.

Suicide Threats

Sometimes students would begin a sentence with, "If I tell you something, will you promise not to tell?" And, I would always tell them that if they told me something illegal or dangerous, I would have to report it. They always told me what was on their mind anyway. Often, what they told me was something like they thought they might be pregnant.

I had several students who told me they were feeling suicidal and I was able to refer them to counseling for assistance. None of them followed through with suicide while I was there. (However I heard later that one of the students I had known did commit suicide a number of years after high school.)

Ongoing Friendships with Former Students

Several former students from the high school are still my friends today. *They are all retired now.* One of them recently celebrated her Golden Wedding Anniversary (Ginger Wood). Now, we are getting to the point where some of my former students have passed away. One, Jay Nankivell, was my good friend and also became a close friend and Masonic brother of my husband. Jay was found dead in his home about a year ago. We had just had dinner with him a few weeks before he died.

I am still invited to class reunions. This is weird, because many of the students I have not seen since they were eighteen are now in their seventies. They always welcome me to their reunions and reminisce about their school days. Sometimes, they tell me that I look better than their classmates. It's interesting to see that people's personalities don't change much. The beauty queen is still the beauty queen and the class clown is still the class clown. Many of the students have done very well in their occupations.

A couple people have told me that they "wouldn't have graduated from high school if it weren't for me helping them." That is very rewarding.

SHMIC

I organized a club for students interested in medical careers. It was called SHMIC. (Students of Hopkins Medical Interest Club) We did many things. We toured the University of Minnesota Hospital, the

Mayo Clinic, the Society for the Blind, and several other health-related facilities. We had speakers about medical subjects.

I also taught the students some basic First Aid and rescue skills. As I will mention later, I also taught nursing assistant skills. Some of these kids went into medical careers, but not all. But, we had a lot of fun.

Jay and Ginger were members of SHMIC. Jay also later taught First Aid for me at Anoka Technical College.

Sports-Related Duties

One of my duties was to be available when they made individual face masks for the Hockey goalies. We put straws in the young man's mouth and nose so he could breathe. (They didn't have girls' hockey then.) Flexible fiberglass was molded onto the student's face and we had to wait several minutes until it hardened. Sometimes, the guys would panic during the process. That's why I was there. When I think about it now, it gives me the creeps, but we never had any real trouble.

I did things for other sports teams as well. For example, I was asked to be at wrestling matches, hockey games, and football games, as much as possible, to provide first aid in case someone got hurt. Fortunately, we never had any serious injuries. At Hopkins, we were also expected to usher and take tickets at basketball and football games.

One of the wrestlers (State Heavyweight Champion—Rick Niles), was also an excellent artist. He was one of my buddies. Later, we hired him to paint some signs for our new Dairy Queen in Buffalo. Still later, he belonged to Burl Oaks Golf Club, where we also belonged (so I got to see him again.) He has also passed away.

I went to a basketball game about fifty years after I left Hopkins. (They are now being coached by Ken Novak Junior, who was inducted into the Minnesota Basketball Hall of Fame after thirty-two years of coaching.)

His father Kenny Novak Senior is also in the Hall of Fame. Ken Senior was the coach when I was there and still helps his son coach at every game, even though he is retired. I started across the floor to say hello to Kenny Senior and when I was still in the middle of the court, he yelled, "Rosdahl, how are you?" I was amazed he still remembered my name after such a long time.

Discipline

Some of the boys would get into arguments and one day two boys were brandishing knives at each other in the hall. The Principal came in and asked me to go break up the fight. He knew they wouldn't hurt me, but was not sure they would not hurt him. He may have been right. I was never afraid of any of the students and I never had any trouble.

One of the Assistant Principals had his office next to mine. He was mostly responsible for discipline. He would have the kids who were in trouble wait in the main office and take them into his office, one at a time. Then, he would kick a wastebasket around and make a lot of noise, so the waiting students would think the student in his office was really getting a beating. (Of course, he did not touch them.)

Then, he would escort the first student out another door, so they couldn't talk to the waiting students. After a few times, he had very little trouble with discipline.

One of the high school boys, Bob M, was in the County Workhouse. I don't know why. Visiting him was a very interesting experience, since I had never been to any sort of jail before. Later, I supervised a program at St. Cloud State Reformatory. (Chapter 7)

SPECIAL STORIES

I had many interesting adventures while working at Hopkins. Some of them really stand out in my mind.

Escape from the Psych Ward

One evening Jerry S, one of the high school boys, appeared at my home in Buffalo. At that time, I lived in an old farmhouse out in the country. Jerry had been committed to a mental hospital (Glenwood Hills) by his mother. (It was possible for a person to commit anyone in those days, often without a hearing.)

Jerry was very afraid and determined to get out of that hospital.

He got a friend to smuggle a pistol in to him and he *escaped from the locked psychiatric unit at gunpoint*. He then *stole a car and came directly to my house*. (I never did know how he found out where I lived.) So, here I was, home alone out in the country with this young man who had threatened people with a gun, and crossed county lines with the gun and the stolen car. I was sure the police would be looking for him by this time.

I was not sure what to do. The first thing I said was, "Give me the gun," which he did. Then, I told him we needed to call the police about the car, which we did. I was never afraid of him, because I knew he wouldn't hurt me, but I didn't know what would happen to him. Since I knew the Wright County Sheriff from my previous employment, I was able to explain the situation to him. He was kind to Jerry and talked to the Hennepin County officials to come up with a plan of action. I truly believed that Jerry was not mentally ill and that he had acted out of desperation and panic.

The bottom line was that Jerry's mother was the one who was mentally ill and no charges were filed against Jerry. His mother was hospitalized and he moved to the home of an uncle until he completed high school.

The Serious Auto Accident

One of my senior students (Johnny N) was in a terrible auto accident near the end of the school year. He was in a St. Paul trauma hospital. He had a tracheostomy (breathing tube), an IV (intravenous infusion), oxygen, a cast, a catheter, and several other tubes. One leg was in traction.

When I went to see him, he said he wanted more than anything to go through his graduation ceremonies. I talked to the doctors and got permission to pick him up and take him to the graduation. We wheeled him across the stage in a wheelchair to get his diploma. I then had to bring him back to the hospital immediately after the ceremony. He was thrilled to be able to go to his graduation and is still my friend today. At one of the class reunions, Johnny was there and he thanked me again for helping him graduate.

The Draft Notice

In the fall of 1963, we got a new Assistant Principal. He seemed very young, but was actually exactly my age. This was during the time when young men were drafted into the military. (I imagine he had been deferred because he was a school principal.) One of the other faculty members got a piece of government stationary and we wrote a "Greetings" letter to him, telling him to report for his Army physical on a certain day. We thought he would realize it was a joke, but he didn't. As the day approached, we decided we had to confess, because if he reported for the physical, he would probably be in the Army before anyone realized the letter was a fake.

I had not seen this man since I left Hopkins in 1966. More than fifty years later (in 2017), he joined my church. And, of course, he still remembers me *and the letter*. We can laugh about it now.

Sexual Harassment

In today's climate of reporting sexual harassment, I am also reminded of my Hopkins story. We had a custodian (George H) who was a super jerk. He had eight children. He gave me a ride one night from Alice Smith School to the high school. He tried to molest me in the car on the way. In those days, you just had to handle situations like that yourself, because there was nobody to report it to. I got nasty with him and threatened to call the police, so he stopped. I never accepted a ride from him or allowed myself to be in a room alone with him after that.

The Foreign Car

One of the teachers, Abner Jacoby, had a foreign car. Very few people had foreign cars at that time. When I came to school, his car lights were on. I tried everything, but could not figure out how to turn them off. So, I went into his classroom and told him I had washed his windshield, turned on the heater and turn lights, but could not figure out how to turn off the headlights. He showed me there was a toggle switch on the dash.

Later, my husband and I bought a similar car. The first time I drove it, I was in Arkansas and not familiar with the roads. It was starting to get dark. I could not figure out how to turn the car lights on. The police stopped me.

I told the officer that I couldn't figure out where the light switch was. He couldn't either. He called another officer who also didn't know how to turn on the lights. Now, it was full dark. A third officer finally figured it out. I was not given a ticket, because the police didn't know any more about the car than I did. (I wish I had remembered the situation with Jacoby's car, because the lights in the car we had bought were operated the same way as those in Jacoby's car.)

Physical Fitness

In those days, there was a great movement in schools for physical fitness. Each classroom at Alice Smith had a chinning bar near the top of the door. One day Superintendent Tanglen, who was about sixty-five, said, "Rosdahl, how many times can you chin yourself?" I figured I could do about two or three. He did about fifteen and probably could have done more.

"The Old Guy"

In about 2000, Joe Rexroad, one of my former students from the class of 1963, called and wanted to meet me for coffee. I had not seen him for about forty years. I asked him how I would recognize him and he said, "I'm the old guy with the cane and the hearing aids." I laughed and said, "Sure, you are." I thought it was a joke, but it was true. He still looked great though and it was nice to see him.

The "Last Twig"

We had a very large family at Alice Smith and their youngest was a student named Twig. I was talking to his mother and asked about the name. She said, "He's the last twig on the tree." Years later, the mother died and in her obituary it listed all her children. And, sure enough, Twig was the last twig on the tree!

Teaching Duties

I was not a regular teacher, but I did have some teaching duties. We had a number of students in the "Work-Study Program." I taught the required classes for Work-Study students in the Nursing Assistant Program. They learned basic nursing skills and then worked part-time in nursing homes to practice the skills. They received high school credit and were employable immediately upon graduation. (Later, when I wrote for Lippincott, I revised the book that we had used in Hopkins.)

I also taught basic First Aid, mostly to work-study and SHMIC students. And, I was in graduate school gaining the education necessary to be licensed as a school counselor, which I did achieve. (Chapter 6) I did some counseling at Hopkins as well.

My " Retirement " from Hopkins

Mr. Tanglen, the Superintendent, retired at the same time I was forced to resign, because I was pregnant. You were supposed to quit at the end of the fourth month of pregnancy. Almost all Minnesota schools had that rule. (See Chapter 7)

My mother had taught in St. Paul and when she was pregnant with me, her yearbook said, "Mrs. Bunker took a *leave of absence for ill health.*" The teachers at Hopkins had a joint coffee party at the end of the year for Mr. Tanglen and me.

When I went in to tell Mr. Coppins, the high school Principal, I was pregnant, he said, "Try to cover it up as much as you can and you can finish the year." (The official policy said you had to quit at the end of the fourth month of pregnancy, "unless they could not find a suitable replacement." They did not try to find a replacement.)

So, I worked until mid-June and had Keith in mid-July. I was enormous by then. Before I started wearing maternity clothes, the students had a bet going as to when I would stop trying to cover up with Pendleton jackets and wear regular maternity clothes. It certainly was not a secret.

When I went into Mrs. Harrison's office at Alice Smith School and closed the door, she jokingly said, "I suppose you are coming to tell me you are pregnant." When I said that was true, she nearly fainted. She really was joking, just because I had closed the door.

Today's School Nurse

School nursing and healthcare has changed a great deal since my days at Hopkins, more than fifty years ago. Many larger schools have a total healthcare team. It is not uncommon to have school psychologists, mental health professionals, social workers, and perhaps a visiting dentist, in addition to a school nurse. (Adapted from *"A Twenty-first Century School Nurse"* in *Minnesota Nursing*, Spring/Summer, 2019)

Today's School Nurse is often expected to give certain medications and/or treatments to students. The nurse refers students to other professionals for special assistance. The nurse also assists in determining which students are in need of items such as free meals or warm clothing.

Most school nurses also make home visits, to assess a student's living situation or to assist the child and family to cope. Paraprofessionals are in the schools to assist disabled students. Nearly all schools also have classes for mentally challenged students and provide special assistance to them.

In today's fast-moving and sometimes dangerous world, the school nurse often acts in conjunction with others to provide grief counseling. This may be during a critical illness or accident, or at the death of a classmate, parent, or sibling.

Schools have special procedures and drills for tornadoes, hurricanes, and earthquakes. Many schools have procedures to be used in the event of a terrorist attack. (*Run, Hide, Fight*) The nurse might be the person designated to organize emergency drills in the school.

When I was a school nurse, I was expected mostly to wait until someone became sick or was injured. Today's school nurse is truly a Public Health Nurse. If this had been the situation, I may have continued as a school nurse. But then, I wouldn't have had all the adventures I had in the Naked City after leaving Hopkins.

My Added Position as a Staff Nurse

My days at Hopkins were fun, but I was bored being a school nurse. I loved the students, but the work was less stimulating than being the County Nurse. In addition, the restraints placed upon me greatly limited what I could do. For example, I could have done more had I been allowed to make home visits.

However, over the years I have maintained friendships with a number of my former students. So, I must have made a difference.

I had already started graduate school while I worked at Hopkins, but I needed something more exciting. In 1964, I started working part-time at Minneapolis General Hospital, in addition to the Hopkins full-time job. I had a chance to practice my basic nursing skills and had many adventures there. (Chapter 5)

That hospital was truly the "Naked City."

To be continued . . .

CHAPTER 5

STAFF NURSE: MINNEAPOLIS GENERAL HOSPITAL

The last two years I was the School Nurse at Hopkins, I was also a staff nurse at Minneapolis General Hospital (MGH). I started in 1964, driving nearly thirty-nine miles one-way from Buffalo. (Minneapolis General Hospital was later renamed Hennepin County General Hospital—HCGH, and then Hennepin County Medical Center—HCMC. The current name is Hennepin HealthCare—HHC.)

This hospital was originally designated as the emergency hospital for Hennepin County. Currently, it is a Level One Adult and Pediatric Trauma Center, mostly for the southern half of Hennepin County.

It is hard to imagine the differences between the Minneapolis General Hospital of the 1960s and today's sleek, modern hospital, with several new buildings and several clinics around the city. The hospital has all the newest equipment and specialized care. It's not the "M.A.S.H. unit" of yesteryear.

The Float Pool

I worked full time summers, as well as part time weekends and school holidays and breaks during the school year. When I was hired, Jane Phillips, the Director of Nursing, told me I would be assigned to whichever unit needed help on a given day. (*I was the entire "Float Pool,"* although that name had not yet been coined. *I was the only floater.*)

So, every day I would call Ms. Phillips and she would assign me to a position. We worked like dogs, but I LOVED it. It was very exciting and I really learned a lot. I worked everywhere in the hospital, although most often I was on Main 3 West, the Men's Surgical Unit. There was great camaraderie among the staff and the patients really received excellent care. *I saw many people walk out of there who would not have survived in another hospital.*

The only reason I quit there was because I was massively pregnant in 1966. And I returned to HCMC later to work in Psychiatry/Mental Health for almost twenty-six years. (Chapter 12)

This was after working more than twenty-five years in education and retiring from Anoka.

The "M.A.S.H" Unit

It's hard to describe the hospital in 1964. We had big open wards, housing twenty or thirty patients. It looked and operated like a military "M.A.S.H. unit." It reminded me of the field hospitals in the Army. Patients had very little privacy, with only a curtain between *some of the beds*. There were no call lights, so patients just hollered "NURSE!" when they wanted help. But, this was a good thing, because the staff could see which staff and which patients needed help. The nurses' desk was closest to the entrance door. (I remember the nurses used to smoke there, if they got a chance to sit down! Smoke breaks were also taken on the fire escapes.)

If we had extra patients, they were lined up in the *middle of the ward*, so they had NO privacy. There were no formal ICUs, so the sickest patients were closest to the nurse's desk. This included patients with IVs, oxygen, suction, traction, casts, circle beds (to enable the patient to be safely turned), respirators (ventilators), catheters and various other drainage tubes. Patients were located further out in the ward, according to their decreasing acuity. The patients on the "porch" were the ones with the least problems. (We did have a *very small* isolation unit—2 North—in a different location.)

It was in one of these wards that the patient described at the

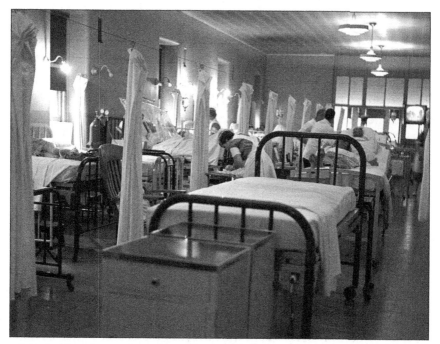

A typical hospital ward in the 1950s and 1960s—patients were close together and had very little privacy (Alamy Stock Photo)

beginning of this book ran down the ward, smashed through the window of the "porch," and ran almost naked into the "NAKED CITY."

The Staffing

The staffing of the entire Men's Surgical Ward usually consisted of myself (the RN), an LPN, and a "nurses' aide."

When I first started, Sandy the LPN working with me, did everything possible to sabotage me. After a few days I sat down with her and asked what the problem was. I said, "We have to work together to care for all these patients. I haven't been here long enough for you to hate me, so what's going on?"

She admitted that she saw my nurse's cap and realized I had graduated from the U of Minnesota. She had been a PN student there and said, "The baccalaureate nurses always got all the good patients." After that talk, we got along fine.

Just an aside: at that time, airline stewardesses were usually required to be nurses. This was Sandy's ultimate goal. However, they told her *she weighed two pounds too much*. She did everything she could to lose the two pounds, but couldn't. So, she was angry about that too.

The nurses' aide I worked with the most was a short, sweet older lady named Jenny. She had worked at MGH for many years. If too many people were hollering for help, she would just turn off her hearing aid, so they didn't bother her. When she retired, she said, "I am going to leave so someone else can have this wonderful job." And, she meant it.

The African American Nurse

If we had extra patients in the ward, we got another staff person, usually an RN. The third nurse was most often an African American man from Chicago, Larry Hill. He was the second male RN I had ever met. (And, being from a small rural community, I had only met a very few people of color in total.) Larry was studying to become a Nurse Anesthetist at Minneapolis School of Anesthesia. We had many adventures on the ward and became good friends. He was very nice and we kept in touch for several years after we both left the hospital. (We wrote to each other while he was deployed in the Army, serving in Viet Nam.)

An unexpected adventure occurred one night when we were driving around about two or three AM (Larry, Sandy, and myself) in Larry's car, looking for a place to have coffee. We were stopped by a police officer, who rudely demanded that Larry get out of the car and put his hands on the roof. (Remember, *this was 1964*.) The officer patted Larry down and questioned him as to, "what he was doing with two white girls."

Then, the officer stuck his head in the car and asked, "Are you girls alright?" We said we were. He asked if we were being kidnapped or anything or if we needed any help and we said, "No."

The officer then asked Larry why he had Illinois license plates on his car, obviously thinking it was stolen. Larry said he was from Chicago and was living in Minneapolis and going to school. The officer slyly asked what kind of school he was going to. Larry said he was a nurse and was learning to be an anesthetist. I am sure the cop had never seen a male nurse before, *particularly an African American man*. (There were very few male nurses at that time and very few African-American nurses.) The officer probably didn't know what an anesthetist was either. He was totally confused and disbelieving.

Eventually, the officer decided he had no reason to hold Larry, so he had to let us go. All in all, I was very embarrassed for Larry and it pointed out how the police sometimes treated people of color. It was a very new experience for me, having always lived in the North. Unfortunately, today we are still witnessing some negative treatment of African American and other people of color in the United States.

On Being Gay

I had met Jonathan M, another African American male nurse, when I was a student at the U. He was openly gay, which was very rare at that time. We did not know anything about gay, lesbian, bisexual, or transgender people. It was a big secret and people rarely "came out." One day Jonathan said to me, "You know, if you were a man, I would love to ask you out on a date." However, that was the end of the conversation.

Then I think back and remember two other good friends who obviously were gay. A close high school friend was named Leo A. People always thought he was "kind of feminine," but didn't think more about it. Later, Leo married a girl named Margaret. I was at the wedding. For years after that, every year I got a Christmas card from "Leo, Margaret, and Vince."

Obviously, these three people were living together. Apparently, Leo and Vince were a couple. I have no idea how Margaret fitted into the group. Later, when Leo died, his obituary in my small hometown newspaper listed Margaret, not as Leo's wife, but as "a good friend" and did not list Vince.

When I was in college, I casually dated Bruce, one of the men on the University's gymnastic team. He was an excellent gymnast and a very nice guy, but I was not interested. Later, he came out and became a very prominent gay activist in Minneapolis. I had no idea he was gay when I was dating him.

The Stabilization Unit

Main 3 West was considered the "Stab (stabilization—pronounced stabe) Unit" for men. If a person came into the Emergency Room (ER) and was going to be treated and released, he or she was handled in the ER. However, if the person was going to be admitted, men were sent up to Main 3 West and stabilized in a small treatment room adjacent to the main nursing unit. (The women's unit was Main 2 West.)

So, if an emergency came up to the unit during my shift, I also had to manage the stab room, leaving the LPN and the aide to run the nursing unit. I remember one time we had two cardiac arrests at the same time in the stab room!

The New Nurse

I always worked the evening shift (3:00 to 11:30 PM).

One day, I got a call from Ms. Phillips about ten AM. "Can you come to work *now*?" A woman had been in a very severe auto accident and had been in surgery for almost twenty-four hours, with surgeons rotating and doing a number of procedures to repair her many injuries. She had multiple bone fractures and other injuries.

When she came up to the unit, she was on a Stryker Frame (to allow her whole body to be rotated as a unit.)

She had Crutchfield Tongs in her skull (to stabilize her neck.) Both legs and one arm were in casts and/or traction. She had a tracheostomy (to facilitate breathing) and was on a ventilator (to maintain her respirations.) She had blood transfusions running in two places, as well as two regular fluid IVs. She also had a urinary catheter.

A new graduate from a small three-year nursing school in Northern Minnesota had been assigned to care for this woman. This new nurse had never seen such a severe trauma case. When I arrived, the new young nurse was sitting next to the bed crying and the nursing supervisor was caring for the patient. I believe the new nurse quit that day; I never saw her again.

P.S. This patient was driving a (fiberglass) Corvette and had smashed head-on into a wall. The car basically disintegrated when she hit the wall. She was a Psychiatric Social Worker.

She was asked several times if she was feeling suicidal and she said, "No, this was not a suicide attempt."

She was in the hospital for a number of months and had many additional surgeries. Sadly, immediately after her discharge, she *attempted suicide again* and this time she succeeded.

Medications

We worked *overtime every day.* Since I worked evenings, I usually came in about 2 PM to set up medications for the entire evening. We had a medication closet in the hall with big bottles of pills and liquid medications and we poured each patient's doses into little cups, using "med cards" for our guides. All the meds were locked in the med closet for use during the shift. We *never had time* to set up meds during the shift. (And always, we were still there until one or two AM, having to complete our handwritten charting after the night nurse arrived.)

Mixing IVs and Calculating Drip Rates

We mixed all our own IVs, adding antibiotics, electrolytes, vitamins, and other materials to them. (Only blood products were set up as they were needed.) We had no IV pumps, so we had to calculate drip rates and dosages. A strip of adhesive tape was placed on the *glass IV bottles.* The approximate run times for the dosages were written on the tape. The nurses had to watch carefully to make sure the IV was running at the correct speed. And if a glass bottle was dropped, *it usually broke.*

Counting Narcotics and other "Schedule" Drugs

All medications for the unit, including narcotics, were kept in the hallway medicine cupboard. (I do not remember if they were double-locked, as they are today.) Each shift, all narcotics and special schedule drugs were counted by the nurse going off duty and the new nurse coming onto the next shift. Both nurses had to sign the drug sign-out sheet. These counts had to match or any missing items had to be accounted for.

If a nurse was stealing drugs for his/her own use, disciplinary measures were taken. Today, medication-dispensing machines do much of this surveillance, keeping track electronically of medications and who is giving them.

Counting Condoms

In those days, condoms were rare. They were sold behind the counter in drug stores and people were embarrassed to buy them. We had condoms, from which we made "condom catheters." We had to lock them up with the narcotics and they were counted every shift. If they weren't locked up, the interns would steal them for personal use. And then, we wouldn't have any condoms left to use for catheters.

Bariatric Care

The Special Bed

We did not have "bariatric" beds, wheelchairs, lifts, or other equipment for very heavy (morbidly obese) people at that time. (Today, most hospital rooms have built-in lifts mounted on the ceiling. Usually, these lifts can handle up to about 500 pounds; some can lift even more. Some hospital beds also have built-in scales, so the patient can be weighed without having to get out of bed.)

We admitted a morbidly obese woman named Martha to the hospital. (The hospital did not have a scale that could weigh her, so her weight was estimated at 450 pounds.) We did not have a bed wide enough to accommodate Martha safely. So, we tied two regular hospital beds securely together and turned them sideways. Then, she was positioned so she was lying *across both beds*. Later, her family brought *her own double bed from home*. (The custodians fashioned wheels for this bed, so it could be moved.)

This bed was safer and more comfortable for her, but it was very difficult for nursing care, because the bed was so low the nurses had to kneel or sit on the floor to provide nursing care. The family had to bring sheets from home, because the hospital sheets were too small to fit the bed.

If Martha required a trip off the ward to the laboratory or x-ray for a test, we had to transport her in her makeshift bed, because we did not have wheelchairs large enough for her. (Bariatric surgery—weight loss surgery—was very experimental at that time and was rarely done.)

Only the freight elevator was large enough to accommodate this lady's double bed, so we had to use that to take her anywhere else in the hospital.

Twinkies

Another *morbidly obese* woman was admitted. Two nurses were giving her a bed bath, carefully cleaning under the huge hanging fat deposits (pannus, panniculus.) Under one of these, was a fully wrapped Twinkie.

When asked about this, the woman said, "Oh, my husband and I play a little game. It's called 'find the Twinkie'!"

When telling about this later, one of the nurses asked, "Was it rotten?" We replied, "No. Twinkies are forever!"

Weight Loss Surgery

During that time, surgical procedures were being developed to assist in weight-loss, many of which were pioneered at the University of Minnesota. (Chapter 2) These surgical procedures assisted obese people to lose weight, although they were not always successful.

"My 600-Pound Life"

This current TV series chronicles the journeys of selected morbidly obese people. Many of them are able to have weight-loss surgery, although they often have difficulty following the restrictions. In many cases, intense psychological counseling is required, in addition to the surgery.

SELECTED STORIES

We saw many very interesting cases at Minneapolis General Hospital, since it was the trauma center for the city. Many very seriously ill or injured people who were brought there survived and returned home.

The Bear Hunter

One day, we admitted a man who had been flown in from Northern Canada. He had been bear hunting and had been shot. The shot had gone through his buttocks from side to side and his butt was nearly separated from his body, held only by a strip of flesh at the bottom. He was just fine otherwise. He thought it was funny (and it really was.) We cared for him until the wound healed slowly—from the inside out—and he recovered completely.

Special Duty

I was assigned as special duty nurse for a very small child who had been beaten by her parents. We cared for her in the PAR (Post Anesthesia Recovery Room), so we would be close to the Operating Room, if necessary. The child was brain-dead and was being maintained by artificial means. The worst thing was that the child's parents were hovering around, looking and acting very concerned. And we knew they were the ones who had beaten her. (Later they were arrested, prosecuted, and served jail time.)

The Girl Who Wasn't a Girl

We admitted a young woman who had been severely injured in an auto accident. She had a woman's name and was wearing women's clothes. We had to cut off her clothes to treat her injuries and when we did, we discovered she was actually a boy. Transgender surgery was unknown at that time and cross-dressing was kept a secret, so this was a surprise.

The Man from the Roof

We admitted an elderly homeless man who was found living on the roof of the Minneapolis Public Library. He had apparently been living there for some time. He was brought into the hospital, because he had a serious wound on his leg.

He didn't want to be in the hospital. "I was doing fine. I could do whatever I wanted. I was able to get food. I didn't have any sex, so when I wanted some, I could sex myself." His leg was treated, healed, and he probably returned to the roof. We never saw him again.

The Tornadoes

On May 6, 1965, a large group of tornadoes hit the Twin Cities area. They took out all the trees around Christmas Lake, west of the City, and demolished a trailer park in Fridley. Many other places were also hit. I called the hospital and asked if I should come in and they said, "Absolutely!"

As I was driving in from Buffalo (about forty miles), I could see tornadoes dip down in front of me and tear things up and then recede back up into the clouds. *I was driving directly toward the tornadoes.* It never occurred to me that I might be in danger. Today, I would be terrified.

Most of the tornado victims were first taken to smaller hospitals, such as Mercy and Methodist. Mercy Hospital had not officially opened yet, but they called in staff and opened quickly to give emergency care to some of the casualties. (The first baby born at Mercy Hospital was born during this time and was named "Mercy." She would be more than fifty-five years old now.)

After stabilization, the more severe injuries were transferred to our hospital. When I got there, the Chief of Surgery, Dr. Claude Hitchcock, was in the driveway telling the ambulances where to go. It was very strange to see such an important man directing traffic, but he did not have anything to do yet. (I ended up staying at the hospital continuously for about four days, just occasionally sleeping a little and then going back to work.)

I was assigned to Special Duty, taking care of two men. One was a Civil Defense volunteer who was hit by a car while he was directing traffic. He had many severe injuries and did not survive.

The other man was an over-the-road trucker. He was found hanging up in a tree, where he was blown by the tornado. His back was fractured and he was paralyzed from the waist down. He survived and went through rehabilitation.

He was retrained to perform some sort of desk job. I talked to him a number of years later and he said, "It was the best thing that ever happened to me. I got an education and now I have a much better and less physically demanding job. And now I am home every night." It was a positive outcome for such a tragic situation.

The Nail Gun Incident

A man was helping a relative with some remodeling. The relative was relaxing up on a ladder holding a nail gun, hanging down. Our client walked under the ladder and accidentally bumped the ladder. This caused the relative to reflexively pull the trigger. The client had a nail totally embedded in his head and brain. Fortunately, no vital structures were involved. The nail was surgically removed and the patient had no after-effects.

Special Situations

Ambulance Runs

At the time I worked at the city hospital, there were three ambulances, which were like station wagons. Two medical interns were assigned to ambulance duty. If the third ambulance went out, I the "float nurse" was assigned to go. I believe that in some cases, I had more First Aid experience and training than did most of the interns.

We had a transponder so we could change the traffic lights in Minneapolis. I thought this was really cool, being from a small town with a *single traffic light* (at the corner of Sinclair Lewis Avenue and The Original Main Street.) Today's traffic lights are preprogrammed to change at particular intervals. The use of a transponder would mess up this programming, so the ambulance just carefully crosses an intersection if the light is red.

There was almost no first aid equipment in the old ambulances and you had to kneel or sit on the floor (in your white uniform) to work with the victim. The ambulance drivers had NO First Aid training. All they wanted to do was load up the victim and get them to the hospital.

The drivers did *no stabilization* before transfer. It was all up to us. So, sometimes we had to fight with them, to keep them from further injuring the victim. Unfortunately, nearly all the interns were men, so the ambulance drivers were more likely to listen to them than to me. I was a young female, so it was harder for me to win arguments with the drivers. (This was basically the same as the ambulance "service" in Sauk Centre.)

Amputated Legs

We were called to treat a twelve-year-old boy who was run over by a train. His body was intact, except both legs were amputated. Since the wheels had cleanly severed the blood vessels, there was very little bleeding.

The boy was very sweet and polite. He said, "Please" and "Thank you very much," which broke my heart. There was no way to reattach limbs at that time. But, he survived, was fitted with prostheses, and did very well. I saw him several years later and he was engaged to be married and was living a full life.

Impaled on a Post

I made a run one evening to discover a man who had been thrown from his car. (Seat belts were not mandatory at that time. In fact, many cars did not even have them.) The victim was impaled on a stop sign post, minus the stop sign. It was the kind of heavy post that is a triangular shape, with bumps on one side. The ambulance driver just wanted to pull him off the post, which was going through his chest.

After a lot of screaming and yelling, I persuaded the driver to wait until someone could come and cut off the pole with a cutting torch, so we could transport the victim with the pole in place. (I knew if we pulled out the pole, the man's lungs would collapse and he would die.)

The man lived after the pole was successfully removed in the operating room. The pole had not hit any vital structures. He had no adverse after-effects from the incident. (It was so unfortunate that I had to argue with the drivers, to avoid further injury to the victims.)

Airplane Transfers

Occasionally, I was asked to accompany a patient who was being transferred to Minneapolis by plane. (The hospital did not have a helicopter at that time.) We flew a small four-place Cessna. In order to accommodate a stretcher, the front right seat and the back left seat were removed. We had one pilot and one nurse on board. The pilot sat in the left front seat. The nurse sat in the right rear seat. The patient's stretcher was placed "kitty-corner" between the seats. A man named John was the pilot I flew with most often.

One patient was over six feet tall and they had not told us that he had a leg in traction, which stuck out about eighteen inches beyond his foot. He had to sit up during the whole flight, so we could get him into the small plane. He had orthopedic surgery at our hospital and recovered nicely.

One transfer was a man from the Dakotas who was coming in for a kidney transplant. This was a very experimental procedure at the time. There were four of us in the plane. (No stretcher was needed.) All the man's wife could talk about during the trip was the plane and how it was her first flight and how exciting it was. I thought it was weird that she did not realize how serious the surgery was going to be. I never heard the outcome of that surgery.

The Earthquake

We made a transfer run to Billings, Montana. We got there late in the evening, so we had to stay overnight. We could only find rooms in a crummy three-story wooden hotel. In the corner of each room, next to the window was a pail containing a rope, which was tied to the radiator. *That was the Fire Escape!*

Also, at the top of the stairs stood two or three pairs of shoes and boots to wear, in case you had to run out of your room without shoes. I doubt if there were any fire alarms and there certainly was not a sprinkler system. I also did not see any fire extinguishers.

My bed was the sort that had just a mattress on top of woven springs. After I went to bed, the bed was shaking and I figured if I could just lie very still, it would stop. And it did. The next morning when we met the ambulance crew bringing the patient to the airport, the ambulance lady asked, "Well, how did you like the earthquake last night?" I had no idea they had earthquakes in Billings! Had I known it was an earthquake, I would have been standing in the middle of the street to get out of that fleabag hotel.

Billings has the weirdest airport I have ever seen. It is up on a plateau. The plane *just drives straight off the end of the flat runway.* Then, it drops down into the valley and climbs up again to reach cruising altitude. It's a shock, if you are not expecting it.

Exciting Landings at MSP

Since Minneapolis-St. Paul (MSP) is a public airport, they had to allow us to land there. The airport preferred not to let small planes land, but they had no choice. We would receive terse instructions from the Control Tower; "Land on Runway 2-9 and *immediately turn right.*"

As soon as we turned, we would see and hear a huge airliner landing behind us on the same runway, going 600 or so miles an hour. If we didn't get out of the way, I guess the huge plane would just run over us. John was an experienced pilot and we always got out of the way very quickly. Again, it did not occur to me to be afraid.

Working Rescue First Aid

As a nurse, I also volunteered to do rescue for the Red Cross, representing the hospital.

The New Baby

One time, I delivered a baby under a tree in Loring Park during the huge Aquatennial Parade, because the ambulance couldn't get through the crowds. We were all done by the time the ambulance got there. The mother and baby were transferred to the hospital as a precaution and everything was fine. (If a baby comes that fast, it is almost always okay.)

The Golf Tournament

I was working a big professional golf tournament for the PGA. I think it was the US Open. A spectator was hit on the head by a golf ball and was unconscious, lying on the ground. The golf ball was lying about a foot from his head.

The Marshal ran up to us and said, "You have to drag him out of the way so the golfer can make his next shot." I couldn't believe it, but he was serious, so we moved the victim.

The golfer was very nice and felt very badly. By the time he got there, the man was regaining consciousness. The golfer apologized and took the man's name. I am sure he sent him a gift. (It is amazing how many people are hit by golf balls at tournaments. They don't show that on TV.)

The Blizzard

We had a severe blizzard and I lived in an old farmhouse about five miles out of town. Four families were stranded for several days, because they had to bring in a special snow scoop to lift the heavily packed snow. One family had horses and one day, a horse walked on top of a snowdrift and fell in. His front legs were on one side of a barbed wire fence and his back legs were on the other side. He thrashed around and was quite badly cut. No veterinarian could get to us, so I was drafted to "fix up the horse."

Several neighbors held the horse and I went to work. I had some penicillin, so I ground that up and threw it into the wound. I took a few stitches with fish line. The only kind of large dressings I could find were some Kotex pads, so I spread them out and taped them over the wound. The whole thing was held in place by an Ace bandage.

The horse completely recovered and did not get an infection. Nurses are always on call! And sometimes, the patients are not humans.

The Small Town Hospital

After I left General, even though I was pregnant, I tried working in a nearby small town hospital. This hospital was basically "owned" by the local doctor. Originally, he had a six-bed hospital in a large house and then the thirty-bed hospital was built by the city.

The doctor was older and ordered everyone around. All the staff people were afraid to argue with him, because they didn't want to get fired. I only had been there a couple days when he ordered me to give an injection of 3.5 Million Units of penicillin to a tiny baby (about six pounds.)

This dose was much too large. I questioned the dose and he yelled, "Don't you dare argue with me!" I refused to give the shot. I quit immediately and refused to come back. I also vowed never to go that hospital for care. Ever.

The Hyperbaric Chamber

The *hyperbaric chamber* (also called the recompression or decompression chamber) is a device that delivers up to 100% oxygen to a patient at greater-than-atmospheric-pressure. (The increased pressure simulates deep-sea diving.) In this high-oxygen environment, in addition to red blood cells, blood and body fluids (including plasma, spinal fluid, and joint fluid), can also carry oxygen. High-pressure oxygen can also trigger healing.

In the 1960s, there were only about eight hyperbaric chambers in the United States and Minneapolis General Hospital had one. So, we got patients from all over the country for treatment. There are now chambers in many hospitals; even a home chamber is available. A mobile chamber can also be delivered to any site in an emergency or as a precaution. Most of the in-chamber staff members in the 1960s were ex-Navy divers.

There are many uses for the hyperbaric chamber. It is often used for deep-sea divers who are down too long or who come up too quickly. (When a diver goes deep, nitrogen becomes compressed by the extreme water pressure and forms bubbles in the blood, replacing the oxygen.)

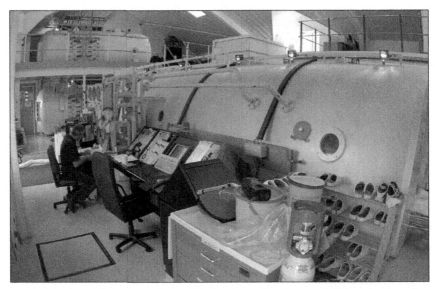

The Hyperbaric Chamber simulated deep-sea diving, forcing the patient's cells to absorb additional oxygen; there were very few such chambers in the country in the 1960s; Minneapolis General Hospital was one location (Sharky/Alamy Stock Photo)

If the diver comes up too fast, *decompression sickness* (DCS, commonly known as *"the bends"*) occurs. This causes extreme pain and possible death. A recent TV episode of "The Curse of Oak Island" used a mobile hyperbaric chamber to treat a diver who had surfaced too fast.

Today, instead of pure oxygen, a mixture of three gases: nitrogen, oxygen, and helium (*trimix*), is often used for diving professionally. This has lessened the incidence of the bends, but is allowed to be used only by professional divers, not by recreational divers.

Other situations when the chamber was used in the early days (and most of which are still valid) were infection with an anaerobic organism, such as gas gangrene (which cannot live in the presence of oxygen) or a gas embolism; sky divers who descended too fast from a high altitude; and cases of carbon monoxide poisoning. In these situations, high pressure (two-and-one-half to five times normal air pressure) allows more oxygen to be delivered to the body.

Today, hyperbaric medicine is also used to treat other conditions, including air embolism, crushing injury, difficult-to-heal wounds or grafts, and anemia caused by excessive blood loss. Some types of surgery may also be done in the chamber. (There also can be adverse side-effects from the high pressure, including pain, ruptured eardrums, or seizures.)

The book, *Manhattan Beach*, describes some of the uses and problems associated with the hyperbaric chamber. (Page 206, in hardback copy, see Bibliography)

Because of the high oxygen content in the chamber, there is great danger of fire or explosion. A number of advancements have been made to reduce the danger. But, the tiniest spark could set off an explosive fire. Staff could not wear any synthetic material, such as nylon (which could cause a spark) and all hair, including facial hair, had to be totally covered.

Special "grounding strips" were worn on the shoes, similar to those used in the Operating Room. Of course, fire danger in the chamber is greater than that in the OR, but it is much safer today than it was in the past.

I wanted to dive in the chamber, but I failed the physical exam because my Eustachian tubes are plugged and my ears won't equalize. I figured this was not such a big deal, so I wanted to dive anyway. They got me down about six feet and I was begging to get out, because of the pain. So I could work outside the chamber, but I could not dive.

Working outside the chamber involves passing supplies, equipment, and specimens through "air locks." These are small separate chambers, with two airtight doors. Only one door can be opened at a time, maintaining the high oxygen pressure inside the chamber.

Working in the hyperbaric chamber was an adventure, kind of like being an astronaut. A little different than regular staff nursing! And it helped to get me an invitation later to attend a launch of the Space Shuttle. (Chapter 8)

CHAPTER 6

GRADUATE SCHOOL AND MARCHING BAND

Admission to Graduate School

While I was the School Nurse at Hopkins, I decided I wanted to also become licensed as a High School Counselor. I applied to the Graduate School at the U of Minnesota. I was told that I had to be a certified teacher and have a minimum number of years of formal teaching experience to become licensed as a counselor in Minnesota, so I was not qualified. I felt my experience as a School Nurse should be equivalent. And, I had taught the nursing assistant courses, sex education, and First Aid. But, I did not have a specific Minnesota teaching certificate. (I was a Minnesota Certified School Nurse, but not a Licensed Teacher.)

I continued to talk to different people in Grad School and they finally got tired of me and said I could "take a course and see how I did." They also reminded me to remember that I *would never be licensed as a Counselor.*" I took the recommended course and got an A. So, they told me I needed to take another course, hoping I would go away. I took the second course and also got an A. Then, they didn't know what to do with me.

I was determined, so they told me I had to take the "graduate record exam." This consisted of several tests, including the Miller Analogies. I didn't even know what an analogy was, but once I got going, I aced it.

Now, *the Graduate School really didn't know what to do with me.* They finally decided I was truly not going away. They told me I could be admitted "on probation." But, they continued to remind me that I could *never be licensed as a counselor in Minnesota* without a teaching license and a specific number of years of teaching experience.

The Graduate School Test Case

After I did well in a few courses, the Graduate School finally relented and decided they would try to make me a "test case" with the State. The Grad School proposed to the State that they waive the specific teaching requirement, because of my unique school nursing experience. *Bottom line*: I did graduate from the program and receive a Master of Arts Degree in Educational Psychology. And I did become the first non-teacher to become licensed as a Minnesota High School Counselor. Furthermore, I now hold a *Life License as a K-12 Counselor*.

The Vocational Education Department

While I was in Grad School in the 1960s, I had to take statistics, which almost drove me nuts, because math is my poorest subject. Some of the guys in Vocational Education were in my statistics class and they helped me through it. I started spending time in the "Shack," a temporary Vo-Tech building on the Minneapolis Campus, because these people were more my friends than the people in the Psychology Department.

In the Voc Ed Department, over the years, I met a number of people who became my friends. These included Brandon Smith, Charlie Becker, Bill Stock, Lloyd Scholer, Mel Johnson, Steve Miletich, and most importantly, Marilyn Cheney (Stern). Marilyn and I were the only women students in the Vo-Tech Department, so we hung around together. And, we were both nurses, the first ever in the Department. (We later did some consulting in the 1970s and taught some courses together.)

One day in the mid 1960s, Dr. Howard Nelson, Chairman of the

Vo-Tech Department, asked me if I would like to teach "Philosophy of Vocational Education" the next quarter. I told him I was not a Vo-Tech major. He was surprised and said, "But I see you around the Shack all the time." Later, I did teach required courses for Vo-Tech teachers for a number of years (Chapter 9), even though I had never taken some of them.

In addition, the guys in the Shack emphasized the importance of *measurable, behavioral objectives in teaching.* This was invaluable when I was writing the nursing curriculum for the Practical Nursing Program in Anoka (Chapter 7) and later when I was writing nursing textbooks. (Chapter 11)

This had never been done in nursing before, at any level.

The EPDA Fellowship

While working at Hopkins High School, I began attending graduate school part-time. I had previously applied for a Federal "Education Professional Development Act—EPDA" Fellowship. I did not think I could possibly win it, because it was specifically for Vocational teachers.

To my surprise, I was named a National EPDA Scholar. By this time I had resigned from Hopkins (Chapter 4), so I was able to attend graduate school. Even though I had a baby son, I felt the fellowship was so valuable I had to take advantage of it. So I started graduate school full-time in fall, 1966. There were EPDA students at Minnesota from several U.S. states including Idaho, Illinois, Michigan, and the Dakotas.

The fellowship paid my tuition, books, and a monthly stipend. I had to take a minimum number of credits and maintain at least a B average. I think Marilyn and I were the first women in the Voc-Ed Department and probably the only nurses in the country to have EPDA fellowships. (It was during this school year that I was approached to start the Practical Nursing Program at Anoka.) I was not supposed to be working when I had the fellowship, but I was also teaching at Northwestern Hospital School of Nursing, a three-year RN school. (Chapter 9)

The Event Leading Up to My Being Hired at Anoka

It was because of Steve Miletich that I was hired in 1967 to set up the nursing program in Anoka. One day, Steve came to me and asked, "Didn't you used to be a nurse?" (Why do people always put it in past tense?) I said I *was still a nurse*; he asked if I had a degree and I said yes. (Thanks to the University School of Nursing.) He said, "I have a friend who is looking for such a person to set up a new nursing program in Anoka. Would you be interested?" Of course, I was. I was interviewed by Howard Rosenwinkel, and the rest is history. (Chapter 7)

Howard had been hired as Director of the new technical school in Anoka *and I was the first person he hired.* (PS: I had some sort of ailment at the time and was in the hospital. Howard came and interviewed me in my hospital bed and he still hired me.)

SPECIAL STORIES

A Consulting Trip with Marilyn

Marilyn and I were invited to the University of California, Los Angeles (UCLA) to consult on the teaching of health occupations students in Vocational Education. First, we went to San Francisco for a couple days. We spent time at Fisherman's Wharf and other landmarks. Marilyn bought a drawing from an artist we met, Scott Sherman.

Then, we drove south down the Coast Road (U.S. Highway 1) to Los Angeles. This road is really creepy for 'flatlanders', because it is very winding. There is a sharp drop-off on the west (right) side and we were tired. If you are going south, which we were, you feel like you are hanging off the edge. I don't believe there were any guardrails at that time.

Our L.A. hotel in Santa Monica was called Hotel Monica. Outside our hotel window was a blinking red neon sign. Part of it was burned out, so it continually flashed "*Hot Monica*" on and off. This struck us as very funny. We enjoyed the consulting trip to UCLA and we learned a lot as well. We also met Diane Watson, who later served with me on the National Health Occupations Advisory Committee for McGraw-Hill and also became a legislator. (Chapter 11)

The Murder Trials

My first husband, Ted, had a cousin (Dick Ross) who was shot. He was staying with Ted's brother, Lloyd. Dick stumbled into Lloyd's house one evening, said either "Lloyd" or "Floyd", and died from a bullet wound in his chest. (I believe he would have lived if Lloyd had known he should plug the hole, so Dick's lungs would not collapse.) The police did an excellent job of finding and extraditing five people from all over the country to be tried for the murder.

One of them was named Floyd, but nobody could ever prove whether Dick had said "Lloyd" or "Floyd." One girl was given immunity and she turned out to be the one who had planned the entire thing. (Dick was flashing a roll of money around and these people decided to rob him. The robbery turned bad and Dick was murdered.)

Long story short, their lawyer was Ron Meshbesher (1933-2018) when he was just starting out, and he was brilliant. He became very well known later and built a very large law firm in Minnesota. The prosecutor for the state was new and inept. Meshbesher made the murderers look like innocent little children and they were all acquitted.

But the greatest thing about this trial was that Marilyn and another EPDA Fellow, Len Brenchley (from Pocatello, Idaho), asked if they could come to the trial with us and we all sat through the entire trial. And, that's where I really got to know Marilyn, who became a very close friend. And, Len was later involved in the "mountain rescue." (Chapter 8)

This was also where I began my lifelong interest in medical forensics and true crime stories. I even did a little legal consulting later.

I was tangentially involved in another murder during that year. I was assigned to interview a young prostitute (actually named Marilyn) as part of a college class. I interviewed her and gave her my calling card. Just a few days later, she was murdered. The police immediately called me in, because she had my card. I was not able to help them much, because I had no idea who might have killed her. It was a very sad case, because she had a small child and was trying to get out of the "business." Unfortunately, her pimp did not want her to quit. I am not sure what happened later or if the perpetrators were ever found and tried.

The Sociology Story

While in Graduate School, I decided it would be fun to take some non-required courses. One of these was a graduate Sociology class. When I got in there, I discovered that all the other students had taken many other Sociology classes. They knew all the famous people and all their theories. Like a dummy, I went ahead and took the Mid-Quarter exam. I failed miserably. Now, I was in big trouble. It was too late to drop the class and I absolutely could not have an "F" on my graduate transcript!

So, I went to the Professor to beg for help. We made a deal. He said he would assign a teaching assistant to tutor me. And, he guaranteed that if I worked hard, I would get at least a B. But, in exchange for this favor, *I had to promise NEVER to take another Sociology course.* ☺ So he furnished a tutor, I got a B, and I never took another sociology course!

Marching Band

Women in the Marching Band

I always wanted to be in the Minnesota Marching Band. (This was one of the reasons I went to the U of Minnesota.) When I was a freshman in 1955, the band did not allow women to march. I was in the band for two years at that time, playing in concerts and pep bands and doing tasks such as directing traffic on Band Day, organizing music, washing spats, and polishing tubas. I can't believe I actually did that. Today's women certainly would not perform those tasks.

Times have changed. In 2006, the first female Drum Major at the U, Molly Watters, was chosen.

In 2016, Minnesota hired the first female Marching Band Director in the Big Ten, Betsy McCann.

Another woman, Emily Threinen, was appointed overall Director of Bands at the U.

We've come a long way, Baby! Thank you, Title IX. Title IX was part of the Federal Education Act of 1972, which stated, *"No person . . . shall, on the basis of sex, be excluded from participating in [any] activity receiving Federal financial assistance."* This included all public educational institutions. This rule also encouraged the development of many women's sports. (NCAA. org, 2015)

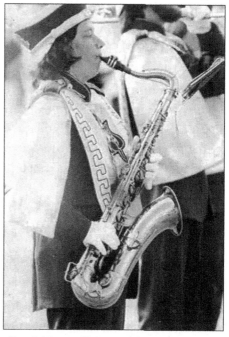

Rosdahl as a 38-year-old member of the University of Minnesota Marching Band (BH Media, MinneapolisStar/Tribune)

Joining the Band as a Graduate Student

In 1975, I took a Sabbatical leave from Anoka and went back to Graduate School, to work full-time on a PhD in Vocational Education. (I did all the course work, but did not write the thesis because by then, I was totally absorbed with writing nursing textbooks.) I decided to join the Marching Band. They had admitted women a couple years earlier. (About half of the band now is made up of women. And, some of them are nursing students. Remember, the School of Nursing would not allow me to be in the band.)

I had played in the band, but had always wanted to march. My graduate advisor, Dr. David Pucel, was looking over my registration and asked, "What's this Music 101?" I told him it was Marching Band and he said, "You can't do that. I think you'll have trouble. My daughter was in the Marching Band and she said it was really hard work." (He didn't dare say he was thinking I was too old.) Marching Band *was very hard work.* After a few days, I was exhausted and stiff and sore. Then, in talking to the other members of the Band, I found they felt exactly the same way. So, I wasn't too old.

"Not Appropriate for a Professional Administrator"

When I joined the Marching Band, I knew if I continued to play clarinet, as I had always done, I would not have a very good chance of being chosen for the marching block, because so many clarinets were trying out.

Since this was my one and only chance to march, I decided to switch to saxophone. I borrowed a sax from a friend and called another friend and said, "Tell me the fingering for something and I will figure out the rest."

He asked me what type of sax I had and I said, "It goes from my knees to my nose." He exclaimed, "That's a tenor. You can't play that. It's too big!" But that's what I played.

I joined the concert band spring quarter of 1975, just to see if I could still play. Then, in the fall, I auditioned and made it into the marching block for football. The Minneapolis Star Tribune did a front-page feature story on me, because I was the oldest person who had ever been in the Marching Band (age thirty-eight.)

Immediately, I got a call from Lew Finch, Superintendent of the Anoka-Hennepin School District, which included Anoka TEC. He told me it was "not professional" to have a school administrator, especially a nurse, "marching around with a bunch of kids. It's embarrassing.

"And, furthermore, we are paying you to go to school." (About 2008, I saw Lew when I was playing for a tailgate event at the Minnesota-Iowa football game. He said, "I see you are still marching around with the Band." He was much friendlier at this point.)

Dr. Ben's Concerns

Dr. Frank Bencriscutto ("Dr. Ben"), Director of the Marching Band, was not happy about being forced to have women in the band. And especially an older woman. He was concerned that I would either

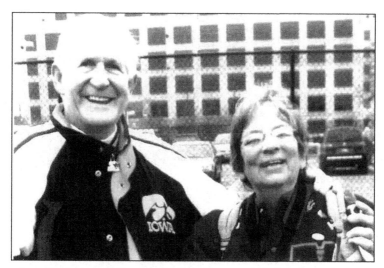

Lew Finch, former Superintendent of Anoka Schools with Rosdahl,
about 2008 (BH Media)

cause trouble or collapse on the field. I did neither. I just wanted to
march.

After each practice or game, he would come up to me and ask,
"How are you doing? Are you okay?" Dr. Ben [1928-1997] was Director of Bands and Professor of Music at the University of Minnesota for
thirty-two Years. He wrote compositions for band and received many
awards. As it turned out, he was less than nine years older than I was.
(University of Minnesota Band website)

Concerns of Counselors at Keith's School

At one point when I was in the Marching Band, we went on an alumni trip to an out-of-town football game. My nine-year-old son Keith
was able to go along. Soon after we returned, I got a call from Keith's
school. "We need to have a meeting with you." I asked what had happened and I was told that I needed to come to the school to discuss it.
I asked, "*What did he do?*" and they wouldn't tell me on the phone. I
was really concerned.

So, I went to the school and was escorted into an office for the meeting. Present were the principal of the elementary school, the school

counselor, Keith's teacher, and the school nurse. They said they had concerns about Keith's mental status. So, I asked, "*What did he DO?*"

"Well", they said, "Keith says you are in the Marching Band at the U." I said I was. (Apparently, they had not seen the newspaper article.)

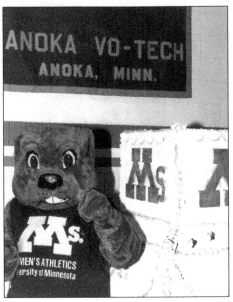

Then, they said, "He says he went on a trip with the University Band." I said that was true.

Then, their final concern, "He says he had a gopher for a roommate." (Obviously, they had never seen the team mascot, Goldie Gopher.) When I said this was also true and explained about Goldie Gopher, they looked chagrined and embarrassed. They had been about ready to send Keith to a Psychiatrist. (Later, I appeared as Goldie Gopher at an event at Anoka TEC.)

Rosdahl as "Goldie Gopher" at an Anoka Technical College event (BH Media)

The "Team" Nurse

But you ask, how is Marching Band related to nursing? A couple years after I was in Marching Band, they were planning a trip out of the country. I asked if I could pay my own way and go on the trip. Dr. Ben said they had never allowed non-band-members to travel with the band. Then Dr. Ben asked me, "Didn't you used to be a nurse?" (There's that past tense again.) When I said I was, he said I could go along on the trip if I would be the "team nurse/First Aid person." Of course, I wanted to go.

Mexico City

We went to Mexico City in 1978 and I was able to take my son Keith, then twelve-years-old, along. The children in Mexico had never seen a large mascot, such as Goldie Gopher, the Minnesota mascot. Most of the children were afraid of Goldie. But the people loved the band and followed us everywhere.

The band was requested to do a Command Performance for the President of Mexico within the President's palace. The palace guards were very curious and suspicious about Goldie in costume. They made the student masquerading as Goldie take off his head and they patted him down, to make sure he was not going to be a danger to the President. There were also armed guards standing on the roof all around the area when the band was performing. (We found out later that there had recently been an assassination attempt on the Mexican President.)

The Hotel Fire

One day in Mexico, I decided to go shopping and Keith did not want to go along. I left him in the care of a couple of friends and I jokingly said, "You stay in the hotel. You do not go outside unless it's on fire!" When I returned from shopping, Keith was standing in the middle of the street.

He began yelling when I was about three blocks away. "It was on fire, Mom. Honest, it was on fire." It was true. There was a small fire in the hotel and they made everyone go outside. Otherwise, Keith would have been in BIG trouble for leaving the hotel.

A small First Aid event occurred when Keith got his finger caught in a conveyer belt at the airport in Mexico City on arrival. This resulted in a Band-Aid and a stern warning from his mother.

Bottled Water

Everyone was very careful not to drink the hotel water from the faucets, to avoid getting sick. One day, we ran out of bottled water, so we went down to the desk with the empty bottles, to get replacements. They just unscrewed the caps, filled the bottles from the faucet, and gave them back to us! (And, we had no trouble, except the few students who did not listen to us and had some GI disturbances, explained later.)

Spain and London

A few years later Keith, my second husband Ron, and I also went to Spain and London with the Marching Band. If I had not been the "team nurse," I would not have been able to go on these trips.

Spain

During the Spain trip in 1982, we took a boat trip past the Rock of Gibraltar to Morocco. Conditions there were a shock to my nursing sensibilities. We were in small groups and were closely supervised by tour guides (one in the front of the group and one in the back.)

The bathroom was simply a hole in the floor and they did not furnish toilet paper. We were seated on the floor for lunch and everything was eaten without silverware. (Many of the students also had the experience of riding a camel while we were in Morocco.)

In Spain, Keith and Ron both bought large souvenir swords. We hadn't thought about how we would get them on the plane to fly home. Fortunately however, since we were travelling with the band, we could put the swords in with the flagpoles. So, there was no problem. Being with the band came in very handy.

London

On the London trip in 1984, the band played at a Tottenham Hot Spurs soccer game (European football.) Tottenham is one of the premier soccer teams in Europe. There was a *high fence and a moat around the field,* to avoid fights after games. There was just a small single gate leading to the field and the tubas, drums, and other large instruments had to go in single file. Since the soccer field is a different size than a football field, the band students first unrolled white tapes to indicate yard lines. The crowd thought that was the show and they all cheered. The soccer crowd loved the band so much that after the game, they all cheered and stamped their feet and yelled. So, we had to bring the band back on the field (through the tiny door) and *do the entire field show over again.*

Nursing Duties on the Trips

One of the girls needed sanitary napkins and finding these was a major challenge, particularly since the store clerks did not speak English and she did not speak Spanish or the language of Morocco. I was able to help her with my very limited Spanish.

Another girl had an itchy rash. I had no idea what the word for rash might be. So, I said "pruritus," which is the medical term for a rash or itch, and the clerk knew exactly what I wanted.

On one of the trips, the drum major Dan Kuch, did a flip on the field. His tall hat struck the ground and he landed on his back. We were concerned that he might have a neck or back injury, but he was okay.

In Mexico, some of the students went to a bar and had drinks containing ice, even though we had told them not to do that. The ice had been made with contaminated water at the bar. Some of them got "Montezuma's revenge" and needed treatment for GI disturbances. Other than that, we did not have any health-related problems.

Other Band Stories

Since I have been associated with the band for many years, I have had many adventures with them.

The Birthday Party

Now I am in my eighties, but I have a number of friends from the band who are twenty or thirty years younger. Recently, one of them called me and asked if he could have a surprise fiftieth birthday for his wife at my house. (He knew he couldn't keep it a surprise at their house.) One day, I was talking to a friend my age and I told her I was having a party for a friend who was turning fifty. She said in a very surprised tone of voice, "You have a friend who is fifty?" I reminded her that if we didn't have young friends, we wouldn't have any friends at all.

Advantages of Band

Joining the Band was one of the best things I have ever done. Not only did I make lifelong friends, but I still play in the Alumni Band for University events and in the Summer Concert Band. I have season tickets to home football games and have attended many out-of-town football games and Bowl games. We recently went to Tampa for the Outback Bowl, which Minnesota won. (Big surprise!)

We have played in a Pep Band at some out-of-town events and special events at the University. I often play in a "Picnic Band" that plays for the "tailgaters" before Minnesota Gopher football games. I have also furnished a band for Nursing School events. And, I am a member of a local Community Band.

In 1992, at the 100th Anniversary of the U Band, I was given the "Director's Friend Award." I have spent many years on the Board of Directors for the UM Band Alumni Society and have been its President.

The Disney Connection

A well-known former U of M band member Stan Freese, is a tuba virtuoso. He has been Musical Director for the Disney enterprises for many years. When my son was young, we made a trip to Disneyland in California. The small Disney band marched out and began playing in the Town Square. Suddenly, they stopped and Freese pointed to me and said, "Rosdahl, what are you doing here?" Band members, as well as nurses, are everywhere!

A ("Medical") Marching Band Story

In the summer, the Alumni Band marches in the mile-long Minneapolis Aquatennial Parade. One year, a few days before the parade, I stepped in a hole and pulled muscles in my right leg and ankle. It was very painful, so I went to a medical doctor. He put it in a cast and told me to be non-weight-bearing and to use crutches for a couple weeks. When the cast came off, I was scheduled to have rehabilitation, to restore the strength in that leg. After about a day, the cast was driving me nuts. It itched and seemed too tight and it was heavy. And, I knew I couldn't march with it.

I knew Fred Cox, the kicker for the Minnesota Vikings. (He was the Vikings' leading scorer for several years.) He was also a chiropractor. I went to see Dr. Fred and asked him to pretend that I was a football player and to tape up my ankle so I could march in the parade. He removed the cast and taped up my ankle. Now, I was able to bear weight and to march in the parade. And I didn't have to have any rehabilitation later. The MD would have been surprised (and probably angry.)

Three Generations at Homecoming
In 2018, my eighteen-year-old twin granddaughters, Emily and Bailey, joined the Minnesota Marching Band. This was, of course, very exciting for me. My son had been in the Band for three years when he was at the U. Now, his daughters were in the Band. So, at the Homecoming Games, *we have three generations of Rosdahls on the field.*

My son is in the Alumni Band and I bring out a huge memorial drum. A local TV station did a story about the three generations.

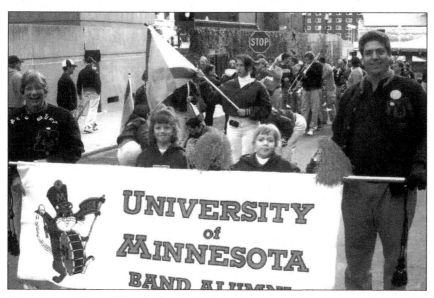

Three generations of Rosdahls march in the University of Minnesota Homecoming Parade, 2007: Caroline, Bailey, Emily, and Keith (BH Media)

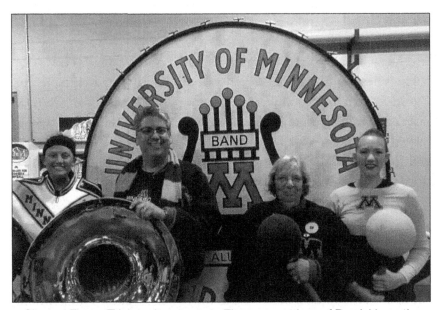

Channel Eleven TV did a feature story: Three generations of Rosdahls on the
field for Homecoming halftime, 2018: Bailey, Keith, Caroline, and Emily
(BH Media)

(Kare 11 Website/Breaking the News/Pride of Minnesota/3 generations. This interview was aired 10-2-18 at 6:30 PM.)

We are certainly not the only family to have three generations of
members in the Band.

But, as far as I know, we are the only family to have three generations *on the field at the same time.* (I am also one of the featured people
interviewed on the orientation film for new Marching Band members.
My granddaughters always get questioned about that. "Is that your
grandma?")

A Final Band Story

When I was small, people would ask my father, "Frank, is that your
little girl?" And, he would proudly say, "Yes."

Then, when I got a little older, my father would say he knew he was
getting older, because now people would ask him, "Are you Caroline's
father?"

Recently, I went to a large School of Nursing dinner and program.

They had five people from the Marching Band come and play a few school songs. (One of them is a nursing student.)

I went up to say hello to the band members and one of them asked, "Are you Bailey's grandmother?"

What goes around comes around . . . .

And none of this would have happened if I had not been a nurse.

CHAPTER 7

NURSING AND EDUCATIONAL ADMINISTRATION

Anoka Technical Education Center

Because I was an RN with a Baccalaureate Degree, I was hired to set up a Practical Nursing Program in Anoka, Minnesota. The original name of the school was Anoka Technical Education Center, "Anoka TEC." The school is now Anoka Technical College. When I started, TEC was part of Anoka-Hennepin Independent School District #11, the largest K-12 school system in Minnesota (37,800 students in 2019), larger than either the St. Paul or Minneapolis schools.

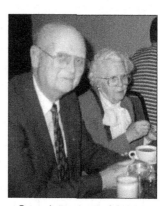

First Days at Anoka TEC

Founding Director: Howard Rosenwinkel

Erling O. Johnson was Superintendent of the Anoka District when I was hired. He had been Minnesota Commissioner of Education from 1961 to 1964. (He signed my first School Nurse certificate.)

Superintendent of Anoka Schools, Erling O. Johnson and Mrs. Johnson
(CB Rosdahl)

133

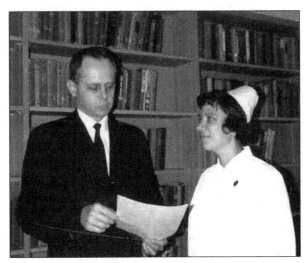

Howard Rosenwinkel, new Director of Anoka TEC, hired
Caroline Rosdahl to establish a Practical Nursing Prog-
am, the first program in the school, 1967 (Anoka TEC)

After his service in the US Army, Howard Rosenwinkel worked
for the Minnesota Department of Education as Supervisor of Vocational-Technical Education under Johnson. Johnson then became Superintendent of the Anoka District and hired Howard to establish a
Vocational-Technical School. Howard served as Director of TEC from
1967 until his retirement in 1984. (Pioneer Press Obituary, March 8,
2015)

Howard was the kindest and brightest man I have ever known. He
had a vision for the school, designing it to be a little different than
other technical schools. He always considered the needs of all students,
without prejudice. He did not see problems, but only "challenges and
opportunities."

Howard was very supportive and would encourage staff to try new
things. There was no punishment if an idea didn't work out. He just
encouraged people to try something else. He was very unassuming. For
example, his desk was a flat door, held up on the ends by two filing
cabinets. He refused to have a regular desk or carpeting in his office.

The building was huge (the largest one-story building in Minnesota), with no internal walls and only a post every sixteen feet. When we

started, the only other people in the building were the secretary, Geneva Johnson; Dick Fries, the custodian; and a night custodian.

First Faculty Member: Caroline Rosdahl

I was the first person hired by Howard on the recommendation of the Vocational Education Department at the University. *Believe it when you hear that networking is important.* Superintendent Johnson was supportive of innovations and I was the *first female administrator in the huge school district.* Establishing a new program was certainly not included in my nursing education, and I didn't have traditional teaching experience. But Howard had faith in me.

I had *only five months* to set up the total PN Program. This involved writing an entire curriculum, hiring faculty, getting the program approved by the Minnesota Board of Nursing, publicizing the program, interviewing and selecting students, identifying textbooks, ordering supplies and equipment, figuring out classroom space, designing a student uniform, and writing contracts with hospitals and other community facilities for student hands-on clinical experience. Other than that, I didn't have anything to do! *Nothing in my nursing education had prepared me for this task.*

The District Administration

Shortly after we started, we shared space with the District 11 Administration, so we saw Superintendent Johnson and other district administrators on a daily basis.

SECRETARY STORIES

Where is my Secretary?

The District didn't think "a woman" was capable of hiring a secretary, so Howard said they would need to supply someone for me. For about two weeks I hauled a big, heavy Selectric typewriter back and forth to my home at night, so I could begin writing curriculum for the program. Finally, I went to Howard and asked about my secretary.

He said, "Don't you have one yet?" He was so busy he didn't have time to think about my secretary. I said I didn't have one and I really couldn't keep dragging the typewriter around and doing all my own typing. I was grateful that I did know how to type. (I had taught myself to type while in high school, having borrowed a typing textbook. I ended up typing the high school newspaper and was Editor my senior year.)

Howard called the District and asked, "Where is Rosdahl's secretary?" Their reply was, "Doesn't she know how to type?" Howard told them I wasn't hired to type and they said, *"Every woman should know how to type!* And, why does a woman need a secretary anyway?" (These were the challenges I faced as the lone woman in a sea of men.) However, I did get a secretary very soon.

Nancy and Colleen

I had wonderful secretaries over the years, including Nancy Bebeau (Zembel) and Colleen Sewell. Nancy was very young when she started. She drove to the school on busy US Highway 10. She was afraid to pull out of the school and cross the highway to merge with traffic. So her husband came every day and drove her car across the road, so she could go home. I could never have gotten the program started and continued without Nancy and later, Colleen.

The Way to File and Type

However, I had some challenging secretaries. One day, I asked my secretary (NOT Nancy or Colleen) to pull out a certain letter that she had filed. She was having trouble finding it and I asked what the problem was. She said, "It's right here in the file. I just have to go through these letters." She had filed *all correspondence "under L for letters!"*

Another secretary had such long fingernails that she had to type and dial the phone with pencil erasers. Those two secretaries didn't last very long.

The Work-Study Student

Early in the program, I had a high school work-study student. I had several specific piles of papers on my desk and I knew exactly where everything was. One day, she decided to "clean" my desk. Unfortunately, she didn't understand my piles and it took me hours to find everything. She was not allowed to touch my desk after that.

A Call from the Governor's Office

Another time, several years later, one of the office secretaries ran breathlessly into my office and loudly exclaimed, "**The Governor's office is on the phone!**" The call was from Herb Johnson, my college roommate's father. Judy had introduced us and I had seen him many times, so I knew him quite well. Herb worked for the legislature. He knew I was a nurse and he wanted my opinion on a person who had been nominated for membership on the Board of Nursing. But, the secretary was very excited to think that the Governor of Minnesota was calling me.

Setting Up the Nursing Program

Developing Course Materials

Developing course materials was a challenge. As a nurse, I had not had much experience with various office machines. (We didn't have computers, or even electronic typewriters, in those days.) It was often necessary to make several copies of each page of a document. In some cases, carbon paper could be used. Erasing was a pain with carbon paper, because you had to erase on each page.

We had a primitive two-stage copier. It's hard to explain, because nobody else remembers it. The typed page was put through the first stage and then that copy (on funny, thin, tan paper) was run through a second time, using another special kind of paper. There were flowers printed on the second paper and it had to be installed into the machine perfectly or it wouldn't make a copy. And, the machine *ate about every tenth copy*! In that case, we would need to type it again. (There was no Photostat or modern copy machine.)

We had a "ditto machine" to make larger numbers of copies, once you typed an original on a special type of paper. The copies got lighter and lighter, the more you made. Eventually, they were unreadable. We also had a mimeograph machine to make multiple copies. The original was typed on a stencil. The drum had to be left in a certain position, or ink ran out all over the floor. (I found that out the hard way.)

Getting Approval from the State and Accreditation from NLN

In order for graduates of any nursing program to be licensed as LPNs or RNs, the program must be *approved* by the state or territory Board of Nursing. (Several of my high school classmates went to a school that wasn't approved and they were never able to become licensed.) The Supervisor of Health Occupations from the State Department of Education, Lucille M, kept telling Howard that I would never be able to get the program approved.

I was following the beliefs of the Vo-Tech Department at the U. and including measurable behavioral objectives in all the course outlines. Lucille also said that behavioral objectives were *inappropriate* in a nursing program, because nobody had ever done them before.

Furthermore, she said they were not appropriate in nursing, because nursing was an emotional and "feeling" occupation and could not be specifically and objectively measured. She definitely did not approve of me writing them and she told Howard this. But, I continued to write the objectives, because I believed in them. (*Bottom line: we did get the program approved.*)

After we began operating, the Minnesota Board of Nursing recognized the value of the behavioral objectives and began recommending our course materials to other schools.

Eventually our materials were used throughout Minnesota, particularly because of the objectives. *These objectives are now used by all nursing programs in the country and those in many countries around the world.* And, the objectives were one reason I was asked to write nursing textbooks. (Chapter 11)

The last I heard, Lucille was no longer with the state and was teaching at another Vo-Tech school (and was most likely using my book containing behavioral objectives.)

Howard and I went to the office of the State Board of Nursing one day. They *actually pulled my licensure exam scores to show him.* This is of course, highly inappropriate and probably illegal. (I was certainly grateful I had passed the exam the first time.)

Later, the National League for Nursing (NLN) also accredited our program. This is a *voluntary national accreditation,* a step above state approval. NLN accreditation is not required, but it greatly adds to the prestige of a school. We were one of the first Practical Nursing programs in Minnesota to receive this national accreditation.

Hiring Faculty

We had excellent instructors. One instructor Lucy Gallese, was to teach Body Structure and Function—BSF (Anatomy and Physiology). She was supposed to write the course outline and it wasn't getting done. So, one day I told her she had to go into a room by herself and do it. She went into a classroom with only a few sheets of blank paper and a pen. She wrote the entire course outline in a few hours *without any reference materials.* And it was perfect. She was a brilliant woman and a great teacher. It just shows that nurses can do anything.

Other early teachers in the program were Gerrie Driessen, Josie Schmer, Mitzi Dee, and Bette Struck. They were all excellent teachers and we worked like dogs. But, we also had a great time.

Bette Struck became Director of the PN Program after I was promoted to Assistant Director of the entire Tech School. By then, I was responsible for all the health-related programs in the school. (Later, I became Vice President of the College and was responsible for *all the programs in the entire school,* health-related and otherwise.) We had added many programs and faculty members by that time.

Admission of Students

Selection of students was another challenge. I visited other PN programs in the state and often found their admission requirements to be *very arbitrary and inappropriate.* All these programs had a *maximum age of thirty-five.* I don't think any programs admitted men. (Several years before, the U of Minnesota had a PN program and they had at least one male student.) Some of the PN schools in 1967 did not admit married students. Out of fairness, I tried to select *the most appropriate students*, ignoring the unreasonable criteria; Howard supported me in this.

We did not have a problem getting applications for admission. So, in our first class, we had a man, Don Yarns. It was quite unusual for men to go into nursing at that time, particularly practical nursing.

Don's case was interesting, because I had taught his wife in the three-year RN program at Northwestern Hospital. When I asked him about his wife being an RN and he an LPN, he said, "She can be the boss at work and I will be the boss at home."

One day, we were talking about emergency evacuation. Don was a big young man. He said I would never be able to move him, so I dragged him down the hall of the school on a blanket. He was convinced and begged me to stop.

We had a number of married students. We also had a number of students older than thirty-five, including one woman who was over sixty. She had to drop out several times for various reasons, but she finished the one-year program in four years, one quarter at a time. (When asked about graduating at the age of sixty-five, she said, "My husband is not well and I want to be able to take care of him.")

At graduation, she had at least twenty-five guests—children, grandchildren, neighbors, and friends. And, she had to commute about fifty miles one-way from Cokato, to get to school.

Another of our first students Betty S, had applied to several schools and not been accepted, because she did not have excellent high school grades. She desperately wanted to be a nurse and I wanted to give her a chance. She was one of our star students and I am sure she continued on to be a wonderful nurse. She eventually became a Registered Nurse (RN).

Supplies and Equipment

Ordering items for the program was very interesting. All deliveries were made to the District 11 warehouse, which was housed in our building. Walt, the Warehouse Manager, got really confused with some of the items that were being delivered. He could not understand why we were getting bedside tables, blood pressure cuffs, and other medical equipment

And other programs at TEC were ordering unusual supplies and equipment. For example, one day Doug an Electronics instructor, ordered a round wall clock for his classroom. When a snare drum in a round box was delivered, Walt took it to Doug. Doug couldn't believe Walt couldn't tell the difference between a snare drum and a clock!

There were many pieces of equipment, which had never been ordered in the school district before. These included electronic equipment and equipment for repairing autos. Later, we had a Farrier (horseshoeing and hoof care) program. Walt couldn't understand why a school needed items like anvils, golf carts, and EEG machines. One day, a truckload of horses' feet for Farrier practice was delivered. They asked Walt where to dump the truck and he thought it was a joke. So, he said, "Oh, just dump it in the courtyard!" Then, people had to get wheelbarrows and clean up the mess.

We received some of our equipment from a nursing program, which had closed, because it was not approved by the State Board of Nursing (so its graduates could never become licensed.)

We got some of our equipment, such as hospital beds, from an Army Surplus place in St. Paul. TEC had an old truck that barely shifted and had very limited brakes. This is what we had to use to pick up things. Some of those trips were very exciting! We also "borrowed" items from the District Warehouse.

The "Kidnapped" Student

We did not have classrooms at the TEC building for some time, because all the walls needed to be built. So, we had to make do with whatever we could find. At first, we borrowed space from Anoka State

Mental Hospital for a PN classroom. We were in the lower level and most of the hospital staff did not know we were there. Since, the PN Program was the first program at Anoka TEC, *nobody had heard of either the school or the nursing program.*

One day, one of our students, Sharon C, was sitting in a lounge at the State Hospital watching TV with several other people. A nurse came in and said, "Okay, everyone. Come on up. It's time for breakfast."

Sharon didn't move and the nurse urged her to come. Sharon said she was a nursing student and the nurse said, "*Sure, you are.* Now, come with me."

Then, Sharon said, "I go to Anoka TEC." And, the nurse said, "*Sure, you do. Come on now.*"

Sharon said, "Our classroom is just down that hall." And, the nurse said, "You are being ridiculous. There is no nursing school in Anoka and we don't have any classrooms here. *You come with me right now or I will call the guards!*" So, Sharon had no choice but to go with her. When they got up to the nursing unit, Sharon was able to convince the nurse that everyone was entitled to one phone call. So, she called me all in a panic and I had to come rescue her.

We had to lock the door to our classroom at the State Hospital, or patients would come in and disrupt the class. I had a work-study student who was afraid, so she locked herself in when she came over there to work.

The "Field Hospital"

We couldn't bring hospital beds, wheelchairs, and other large equipment to the State Hospital, so we had to create a Nursing Arts Laboratory in the empty TEC building. Since all supplies and equipment for the entire Anoka District came into the temporary warehouse in our building, I went there to see what I might be able to use ("*borrow/ steal.*") All the toilet paper for the entire year, for the entire huge district, was delivered in the fall. Hundreds of large boxes. So, we were innovative. We took a bunch of these toilet paper boxes and built walls to provide privacy when our students were practicing procedures like back rubs and bed baths. One of the men in the building went by and said, "This looks just like the M.A.S.H. Field Hospital when I was in the Army." Thus, the Nursing Arts Laboratory came to forever be called the "Field Hospital."

One day one of my instructors Dick Spicer, was wheeling an empty handcart down the hall. Someone said, "I wonder what he is stealing from the warehouse today?" And, another person replied, "Maybe he is stealing hand carts."

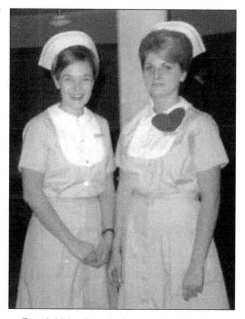

Rosdahl had to design nursing student uniforms and caps for the new program (CB Rosdahl)

Uniforms and Graduate Pins

I chose a basic blue uniform with a white yoke. I had to choose a uniform for Don to wear. But, that was easy. He just wore a blue top that matched the women's uniforms and white pants. Our student caps were plain white, with traditional "wings." (Of course, Don didn't have to wear a cap.)

We had a contest among the students during the year to design a pin to be given

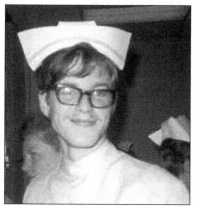

A male student tries on a nursing cap (CB Rosdahl)

to graduates. All nursing schools had graduate pins at that time. You could tell what school a nurse graduated from by looking at their cap and pin. One of the students came up with a very nice design, we contacted Josten's, and the pins were manufactured. (I don't know if they still give out pins or not.)

Clinical Facility Contracts

It was necessary to arrange hands-on clinical experience for the PN students. Mercy Hospital in Coon Rapids was very new and Tom Mattson the Administrator, had been one of the driving forces in obtaining the PN program for Anoka. So, we were welcomed there for clinical experience. In addition, we wrote contracts with Anoka Nursing Home and some other community agencies. Later, we added Unity Hospital in Fridley. I am amazed at how large these hospitals are now. They were very small when we started the PN program.

Lucy Fallon was the Nursing Director at Anoka Nursing Home when we started. She remembered me and was instrumental in my being hired many years later as a Staff Nurse at Hennepin County Medical Center. (Chapter 12) Networking is valuable for nurses, just as it is for others.

FACULTY STORIES

I had a number of experiences while interviewing, hiring, and supervising faculty. I interviewed a new graduate from a four-year degree RN program for a teaching position. I asked about her hands-on technical skills and she said, "I took blood pressure and temperature a couple times. And, I saw a movie on catheterization." That was the sum total of her clinical experience! All the rest of her education was in the classroom or simulation laboratory. She couldn't understand why I wouldn't hire her to teach in our hands-on basic PN program.

I had one instructor who was a "non-recovering" alcoholic (Margaret D.) She came to work several times "under the influence." After several warnings, I had to let her go, even though she was a good teacher. (She later married the Director of a chemical dependency treatment center.)

I hired another teacher (Yvonne S.), who was also unable to stop drinking. She went through treatment and was later hired as a Head Nurse at a local hospital. She later told me, "Getting fired was the best thing that had ever happened to me, because I got my life together." She thanked me and we became friends.

One of our other instructors left her husband when she learned he was having an affair *with* another man. They reunited and separated several times after that.

Dick Spicer

Dick has been mentioned before. He was a very popular instructor. He was very quick on the comeback and always had a joke. One of the most interesting things about Dick occurred when I first interviewed him for his position. *I had never met him.* He wanted to be my assistant, responsible for the health-related Secretarial programs. On the evening he wanted to be interviewed, I did not have a babysitter for my son. So, he agreed to come to my home for an interview. He then asked, "Do you have a washer and dryer?" I said I did, so *he brought his laundry to the interview.* (I don't suppose that would be allowed today.)

Developing Additional Health-Related Programs

I was Director of the Practical Nursing Program and taught in the program for the first year. The next year, my assignment was to start other health-related programs. Within a few years, we had a number of these programs, including Nursing Assistant, Human Services Technician, Occupational Therapy Assistant, Physical Therapy Assistant, Respiratory Therapy Technician, Surgical Technician, and EEG Technician. We also developed a number of health-related secretarial programs including Medical Secretary,

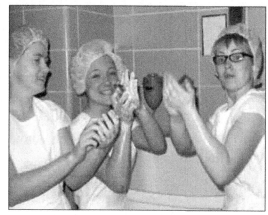

Handwashing practice for health occupations students (CB Rosdahl)

Medical Record Technician, and Hospital Station Secretary. I had overall responsibility for all these health-related programs. And, I learned a lot about all these occupations.

Cooperative Programs with local Colleges

During the early years, we built a one-plus-one nursing program with Anoka-Ramsey Community College. This program allowed our graduate LPNs to go to school for an additional year and become two-year RNs. (This model has now been developed elsewhere in Minnesota and the U.S.) We also cooperated with two-year colleges for other Associate Degree programs, such as Occupational and Physical Therapy Assistant; and Respiratory Therapy, Medical Record, and EEG Technician.

Added Responsibility for Additional Programs

At first, my title was *Assistant Director* of Anoka TEC. This title eventually evolved into Vice-President of Anoka Technical College. By the time I left, *I was responsible for all the programs in the college.* This included Automotive Occupations, Cooking and Baking, Landscape Careers, Electrical and Electronic Careers, Office Careers, Drafting, Building Trades, Aviation, Apparel Specialist, Welding, Farrier and others. I had many adventures with these programs. And, I learned a lot about occupations that as a nurse I had not been exposed to before, such as Air Traffic Control, Electrical Design, and Golf Course Management. These experiences, of course, are not in the life of a typical nurse. They created many interesting adventures.

One day, the Golf Course Management teacher called me all in a tizzy. He said, "One of the kids drove the bobcat into the creek!" I know he thought I would be angry. I thought it was funny and asked, "Don't bobcats know how to swim?"

One of the program instructors had a boat on Lake Minnetonka. The boat was named "Intern-Ship." So, if he wanted to take the students out for a fun day, he would say, "We are going out on internship." I knew where they were going, but nobody else did.

146

One of the male instructors Wolf, a staunch German, was very angry when I became his supervisor. He didn't want to work for a woman. So, I sat down with him and said, "You know, it's kind of like a *shotgun wedding*. You are stuck with me and I am stuck with you." After that, we got along fine. As an ironic twist, *my son married his niece. So, now I call him "Uncle Wolf."*

Special Cooperative Programs

In addition to cooperative programs with community colleges in the Twin Cities, we had cooperative programs in other areas of the state. For example, we had a cooperative Surgical Technician program in Duluth, Minnesota. I had to travel up there occasionally, on the shores of beautiful Lake Superior to visit the program, although my faculty handled most of the details.

Probably the most interesting cooperative program for me was the Baking Program at St. Cloud State Reformatory. I had never been to a maximum-security prison before, so it was quite an experience. I learned things such as why inmates were limited to five slices of bread at meals, (because it could be used to make "hooch.") The thing that surprised me the most was that the inmates *were so young*. I had always pictured a prison to be filled with middle-aged or older men. I hope the prison system has developed additional educational programs to assist inmates when they are released.

All these experiences enhanced my ability to be a good nurse and to relate to all kinds of people.

Adventures with District 11 Administration

The Pregnancy Policy

Most school districts at that time had a policy that a female teacher had to quit teaching at the end of the fourth month of pregnancy. This happened to me at Hopkins. (Chapter 4)

The policy was unreasonable. Since we were sharing space with the District Administration, I saw them nearly every day. About the third year of the PN program, one of my instructors, Josie, was pregnant. Assistant Superintendent Cleveland came up to me and said, "You know, that woman is pregnant."

And I said, "You are absolutely right."

He asked what I was going to do about it.

And I said, "I think I will just wait. I believe it will go away."

With Howard's support, we just ignored the pregnancy, even though Cleveland continued to mention it. And, sure enough, it went away. *That broke the unreasonable policy for the entire huge District 11.* Other schools in the state then followed Anoka's lead. Since Anoka was the largest school district in the state, fairly soon the policy no longer existed in Minnesota. I am proud of this accomplishment, because getting rid of the policy benefitted many people.

Several years later, Cleveland came up to Josie and asked, "Did you ever have that baby?" She didn't quite know how to respond, since her daughter was then six years old and in first grade.

The Policy Against Hiring Husband and Wife

Anoka also had a policy stating that husband and wife could not both teach in the district. This was ridiculous, since there were about twenty to twenty-five schools in the district. I understand not having them in the same school, but in that huge district, the policy did not make sense.

I wanted to hire a woman who just happened to be an Assistant Superintendent's daughter and was also married to another teacher in the District (not TEC.) Her father called me and asked, "Were you talking to my daughter about teaching at TEC?" I said I was and he said *I couldn't hire her.*

I asked if she was a licensed RN and he said, "Yes, of course."

I asked if she had a drinking problem. And he said, "No, certainly not."

I asked if she had ever been arrested or had committed a felony and he said, "Heavens, No!"

I asked if she had some mental health problem that I was not aware of and again, he said "No."

He could not think of any reason not to hire her, except it would make him look bad because of the unreasonable District rule. So, again, with Howard's support, I hired her and she taught at TEC for many years. *This broke another unreasonable policy for the Anoka District that needed to be broken.*

Later, I married one of the TEC teachers. This was clearly against District policy, particularly since I was his Supervisor. We eloped and did not tell anyone we were married for some time. We then talked to Howard and he did not have a problem with us being married. So, we continued to work together for a few years, without any repercussions. (I left several years before he did.)

FAVORITE STORIES

The Cut-Up Car

An older car was parked in the school parking lot for a long time. It appeared to be abandoned. One day, the Automotive Instructor Jerry, told a couple of students to practice their skills with the cutting torch and go out and cut up that old car. This was a great idea, except *they cut up the wrong car!*

I got involved because the cut-up car belonged to one of my nursing students, Patty M. So, the nursing instructor and I had a big meeting with the Counselor, the Chairman of the Automotive Program, the student, and her husband. Patty thought it was funny. Her husband did not. She tried not to giggle during the meeting, but was not very successful. We quickly resolved the situation, but it will always be remembered by those who were there. It's a TEC legend.

Clinical Dress Code

Some of the students wanted to wear their uniform skirts very short (in style at the time.) They were allowed to wear white pants and a top like Don's, but some preferred skirts. I talked to them about what would be visible if they bent over a bed in a short skirt. My words fell on deaf ears. So, one day, I took my camera with me and shot photos from the back when students bent over. Then, I posted these photos on the bulletin board at school. You could not see anyone's face, just her underwear. Students came in and looked at the photos in shock. "Is that me?" I did not have any further trouble with short skirts.

Blue Hair

One of my instructors, Gerry, came to me one day and said, "I have a student who came to school today with bright purple hair and we are supposed to go to the nursing home tomorrow. I'm afraid some little old lady will have a fit. I don't know what to do." (Remember, this was in the early 1970s when people didn't have brightly colored hair.)

I asked if the student's work was okay and Gerry said it was. So, we decided there was nothing we could do except let the student go to the nursing home.

The next day, the student walked into the room of an elderly lady. The lady exclaimed, "Oh! How do you get your hair that beautiful color? *Mine always turns blue*." (So, it was not a problem.)

"It's Mine Today!"

We had a student named Mario, from Mexico, who spoke very limited English. He was habitually late or absent. The instructor told him they were having a test the next day and *he had to be there and be on time*. He said, "I will be here." The next day came and Mario didn't. He showed up about two or three hours late.

The instructor asked where he had been and he said, "I did not have a ride."

She asked, "So, how did you get here?" Mario said, "I stole a car."

The instructor said, "You can't just steal a car. Whose car is it?" And, Mario said, "*It's mine today!*"

The instructor said, "But you don't even have a driver's license." And, he said, "I have my mother's."

The instructor came to me and told me the story. She asked if she would be in trouble. I asked, "Did you steal a car?" When she said no, I told her it was not her problem.

About two weeks later, Mario came into my office leading a young girl. He said, "This is Anita. I give her to you." In shock, I asked what he was talking about. (What he intended was to have Anita take the Nursing Assistant course.) But, his first statement was a surprise.

The Painter

We were often under construction in the early years. One day, Lucy was teaching a class on childbirth and a painter was painting the wall in the back of the room. Lucy told the class she would be showing a movie about childbirth.

Part way into the class, she realized that the painter was going up and down with the paintbrush, but hadn't moved over for several minutes. She asked him if he had a question and he said, "I have several children, but I have never seen a delivery." So, she invited him to sit down and join the class for the movie and he thanked her profusely afterward.

The Omission

I had an instructor who was an older, very proper, single lady. About the second year of the program, I was talking to one of her students and the student asked me a basic question about the Reproductive System. I answered the question and then asked her if she didn't remember that from her anatomy class.

She said, "Oh no. We don't study the Reproductive System in that class!"

To my horror, I found out that the regular instructor was too embarrassed to teach that material, so she just omitted it. So, we had this material taught by another instructor, to make sure it got into the program.

The Concert

In 1971, some of the students decided they wanted some sort of program at school. One of the girls in nursing had met a new singer who had performed at her high school (Edina, Minnesota). She said he was really good and was trying to make it in music. So, I contacted him and he agreed to do a concert for us. He said the charge would be $50. We agreed to this on the phone. We had a verbal agreement (no written contract or even a handshake.) I had not personally met the man.

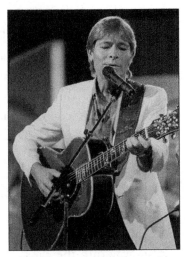

John Denver gave a concert in Anoka, Minnesota in 1971 (Gisjbert/Alamy Stock Photo)

Before the date of the concert, this singer *John Denver* released his hit song, "Country Roads." He became an overnight star. Denver still came and did the concert for TEC and *we paid him $50*. He was a real gentleman. And a great singer.

Several years later, I was in Arkansas and I was looking at the local community bulletin board. There was an ad from a lady saying, "I am selling my home and my furniture and moving to California to live with my son, John Denver." Unfortunately, he had just been killed a few days before that. I have no idea what ever happened to his mother.

Miss America

Gretchen Carlson from Anoka was Miss Minnesota in 1988 and was named Miss America in 1989. She made several visits to TEC. (She later became an advocate for women's rights in the U.S.) Our Director at that time (not Howard) was very awed by her. She was

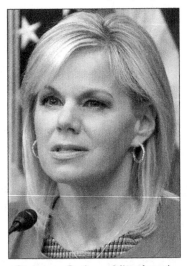

Gretchen Carlson, Miss America-1989, made several visits to Anoka TEC (Wikimedia)

very impressive, as well as beautiful and gracious. And, she has done very beneficial things for the U.S. She has written several books, including BE FIERCE and GETTING REAL and has been profiled in movies including "Bombshell" and "Persecuted." (Google, 2019; see Bibliography)

The Teachers' Strike

One year, the teachers in the District went on strike. Since we were part of the District, our teachers were expected also to go on strike. This presented problems for some students who had specific completion dates for their education or who had already accepted jobs. Therefore, a few of the TEC teachers crossed the picket lines and continued teaching. Unfortunately, the striking teachers were very angry about this. (The people who crossed the picket lines were ostracized and the other teachers ignored them later.)

I was an administrator and was married to a teacher. Howard, the Director, called me in and asked me not to ride to school with my husband, because he was on strike and I wasn't. (Being a smart aleck, I asked if it was okay for me to *sleep with him*!) So, we had to drive separately. Since we lived twenty-seven miles away, this was an inconvenience.

The Organ Trial

There was a party one evening. I had just hired a new instructor, Fred. Since he was so new, I didn't know anything about his life. In the middle of the party, he dragged me outside and said, "You have to leave with me, because Susan is hustling me and I am gay and I don't know what else to do." (This was long before gay people were coming out.)

I told him I didn't care if he was gay, but if he propositioned any student he would be fired because of the customs and rules at that time. I knew the District would not allow him to stay. One day, a tough Army veteran in Fred's program came into my office, slammed the door, and began to speak. I did not need to ask what was bothering him. So, Fred agreed to resign.

However, Fred had taken a loan from the school Credit Union to buy an electric organ for his home. He refused to pay them back and when the District asked for their money, he said, "Rosdahl told me I didn't have to pay it back, because I was fired." Of course, I had no influence over the Credit Union, so this was untrue.

We went to court with the Credit Union's attorney. And, the District furnished me with an attorney. My attorney was a very new Law School graduate and he began trying to make deals with Fred and his attorney. I took the new young attorney out in the hall and asked what was going on. He *began to cry* and said, *"I have never been to court before and I don't know what to do."* (I found out that courtroom practice was *an elective course in law school.*)

I told the lawyer not to say anything else and I would handle the case before the judge. We resolved the case and the money was paid back. Little did I know *I would also be a "pseudo lawyer"* during my nursing career.

Ten Most Wanted

One of my instructors was watching the TV program "Ten Most Wanted." This program showed photos of criminals wanted by the FBI. She saw the photo of a patient she had seen in the hospital. She called the FBI and they arrested the man without incident.

The Request for a Nursing Student to Work

When I was in high school, we had an administrator who was sexually inappropriate with teen-age female students. I am sure he actually molested some of them. There was nothing that could be done about this at the time. It would be the student's word against the man and no doubt, the court and/or police would believe the "important" administrator. (I believed the story was true, because he had tried to molest a good friend of mine and I truly believe the story she told me was absolutely accurate.)

To make matters worse, this man's son was later arrested in Minneapolis for luring young girls to a hotel room and promising to make them movie stars. He then molested the girls and distributed pornographic photos of them. He threatened them, to prevent them from reporting the incidents. But, fortunately, he did get caught and prosecuted.

So, early in my career at Anoka, I received a letter from this former school administrator (the father) who now lived in the Twin Cities area. He asked if there was a nursing student who would come to his home and help care for his wife who had suffered a stroke. There was no doubt that the letter was from the same person who had worked in my high school. I immediately recognized his name and his very distinctive signature.

Of course, he had absolutely no idea he was writing to me, because the letter was just addressed to the "Director of the Nursing Program." In addition, my name had changed because I was married. It was a great pleasure to write back to him and tell him that I would not allow any girls to work for him. Ever. I am sure he almost died of shock when he saw my signature on the letter. I know he realized who I was. And, he probably knew I was aware of his history. *Sometimes, there is justice in this world.* And, if I had not been involved in nursing education, he may have obtained another young woman to molest.

The Blind Student

I got a call one day from a Vocational Rehabilitation Counselor. He said he had a blind girl who wanted to be trained as a Surgical Technician. I asked if she was totally blind and he said she was. He said she had a trained Guide Dog to help her.

I told him I couldn't imagine how she could be a Surgical Technician. She would have to thread needles, anticipate and choose appropriate instruments for the surgeon, prepare and label specimens, and measure liquids and medications. And, there was no way that a dog would be allowed in the Operating Room.

He couldn't understand why some sort of special arrangement could not be made for this student. He thought she could be specially trained. So, we set up a mock Operating Room at the school and invited the student and her counselor (and her dog) to come in. We then had her try to do some of the tasks. Unfortunately, she was unable to do them without her sight.

The girl realized that her goal of becoming a Surgical Technician was not reasonable. She then chose to become a Medical Secretary and Transcriptionist and she did very well.

I am still picturing a dog in a little green suit, wearing a cap and face mask, working in the Operating Room!

The "Sick" Rabbit

We had a student in one of our programs who had serious mental health issues. He was quite well controlled when he took his medications. However, when he didn't take them, he had many problems. His wonderful and caring instructor Gerry, called him every morning and asked if he had taken his psych meds. And, if he hadn't, she would tell him to go take them. (She had informed him that he would not be allowed to come to school unless he took his meds.) He remained able to function as long as Gerry called him daily. She even called him on weekends.

One day, Gerry could not locate the student. We found out that he had a pet rabbit. That day, the rabbit had died. He had taken it to the Emergency Room at Mercy Hospital. When they told him that they didn't take care of animals and there was nothing they could do, he refused to leave. He could not believe the rabbit was dead.

The young man was causing a lot of trouble and had been throwing and breaking things. They were unable to reason with him and had to call the police. The young man was taken to a Mental Health Unit for treatment. I don't know what finally happened to him, but we were unable to allow him back into the program for safety reasons. (This episode was a good introduction to my later work in Inpatient Psychiatry.)

Selected Faculty

Elaine Koivumaki

Several years after the school was started, Elaine another Supervisor at

TEC, was walking out to her car in a rainstorm carrying an umbrella. She was struck by lightning and killed instantly. It was very sad, but a good lesson for all of us. *Do not carry an umbrella with a metal handle in a thunderstorm!*

Gen Olson

Gen was one of the Supervisors at TEC. She later took a Sabbatical leave to attend school. After her year off, she told the new Superintendent Lew Finch, that she did not plan to return. He told her she would have to pay back the money from the Sabbatical. She said that was no problem and she paid it back. Finch said to her, "You are making a big mistake. You will never find another good job like this."

However, Gen became a very influential Minnesota State Senator (1983 to 2012—over 10,000 legislative days.) She was

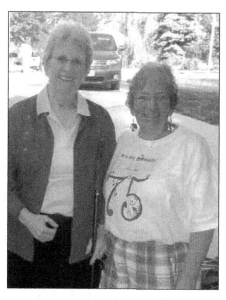

Rosdahl and former Minnesota Senator Gen Olson, 2012 (BH Media)

Chairman of the Education Committee, so she helped to make policies, which directly affected the school (including policies related to funding.) She greatly helped advance the cause of education in the state. And, I would imagine the Superintendent reconsidered his words about her being able to find another job.

The New Director

In the fall of 1984, after Howard retired, the school hired a new director, Ahmed H. He was from Pakistan and was NOT happy to have a female assistant (me.) One day, Ahmed hit me. I went to one of the District Administrators, and his response was, "Oh, Ahmed was just kidding." He was *not kidding*, but that was the type of support women got in those days. Harassment was just part of the job and you had to deal with it yourself. So, the second time the man hit me, I said, "If you ever touch me again, I will call the police and file charges."

So, he never hit me again, but we had a very difficult relationship. He did not get along with many of the staff and faculty. Things were very bad and he was finally asked to leave in 1988. *We were not taught how to handle situations like this in nursing school.*

Years later, I saw this man's wife, who is a well-respected physician. I asked how Ahmed was. She replied, "I don't know and I don't care." So obviously, they were no longer married. I don't believe Ahmed ever got another job in Vocational Education.

National and State Involvement

American Vocational Association (AVA)

During the time I was at Anoka, several of us became involved with AVA. I went to several national conventions and was on some national committees. This was very interesting and I learned a lot. I was able to meet vocational instructors and administrators from all over the U.S. I especially got to know the health-related instructors from the University of Iowa. They included Milf Rosendahl (who some people thought was my relative—she wasn't) and Dale Peterson. Dale was interesting, because he was a Professor at the University during the school year and a *rodeo cowboy during the summer.*

Membership in AVA eventually led to my appointment to a National Advisory Committee on High School Health Careers for McGraw-Hill. (Chapter 11) This committee was very important in my nursing and writing career.

Minnesota Vocational Association (MVA)

I also belonged to the Minnesota affiliate of the AVA. I held several offices in this organization. Early in my career at Anoka (1969), the MVA established a new award for outstanding service and leadership in

Health Occupations Vocational Education. This award was named for Verna Mae Blomquist, who previously had been the State Supervisor for Health-Related programs. I was the first recipient of this award and it was a great honor.

Minnesota Assistant Director's Association

I was active in the state association of vocational school Assistant Directors and was elected its President. I considered this a great honor, since I was the only woman in the state (and certainly the only nurse) who was an administrator in a vocational-technical school.

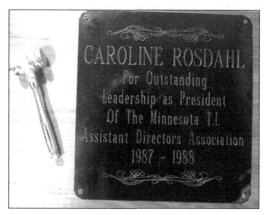

Rosdahl, (first woman AVTI Assistant Director in Minnesota,) received a special award as President of the Association, 1987-'88 (CB Rosdahl)

This association gave us a chance to discuss mutual concerns as a group and helped solve some of the problems facing vocational and health occupations education. I also visited a number of other Vo-Tech schools as part of my responsibilities.

Society of Manufacturing Engineers

I also was a member of the Society of Manufacturing Engineers, because of some of the later programs I supervised at Anoka. This was extremely interesting, because I didn't know anything about manufacturing engineering when I joined. Nurses need to be flexible.

An Interesting Footnote

Both my husband Ron and I worked at Anoka TEC for more than twenty-five years. I retired when I hit the "Rule of 90" and got full pension. Several of our children and other relatives graduated from TEC and got good jobs. My son Keith, a graduate of Ron's Electrical Design

Program, is now a full partner and Vice President of Parsons Electric, one of the largest Electrical Construction companies in Minnesota. Ron's son Gary took over RC Consultants, Ron's electrical consulting business, when Ron retired. They have more than ninety employees. In addition, Ron's daughter-in-law, Lynn Christensen, and several of his nephews also graduated from TEC.

If I had not been a nurse with a degree, I would never have been hired to set up the PN Program. I would not have had the opportunity to learn about Vocational Education and about the myriad of careers in business and industry. There are so many types of employment available to nurses. The sky is the limit!

CHAPTER 8

SPECIAL NURSING-RELATED STORIES

I had many adventures that related in part to my nursing experience and training. I feel that I was able to help in some way in these situations.

Automobile Accidents and Other Disasters

Because I commuted about thirty miles one-way to school and also commuted to other jobs, I came upon several serious car accidents. I felt I should stop, particularly if the police had not yet arrived. When I worked for Wright County, the Sheriff would stop me and ask me to help if there was a serious accident.

The Car Explosion

One situation involved a woman and a child in one car who had been hit head-on by an oncoming car. The man in the other car was obviously dead. (There were no police on the scene when I arrived.) The woman in the first car was injured.

It is general practice not to move injured people. However, I felt we had to get the woman out of the car, because there was gasoline running all over. I was afraid of an explosion. A bystander and I gently pulled her out the back window of the car, because the doors wouldn't open. She told me she was sure her child was dead. I went back to check the child and got no pulse. We couldn't figure out any way to get him out of the car. We just barely got out of the way, and the car exploded!

The woman later told me that her child was severely mentally and physically disabled and the doctors had said there was nothing they could do for him. She said, "It was a blessing that he passed away without suffering."

People Thrown out of their Car

Another time my husband and I were driving on a freeway and a semi truck in front of us suddenly slammed on his brakes. We stopped and the scene before us was terrible. A car had crossed the grassy median and struck an oncoming car head-on. The truck had swerved to avoid hitting the crashed cars.

Several people were lying on the road. (No seat belt laws at that time.) They had terrible injuries, but we were able to give them some basic First Aid and the trucker called the police on his two-way radio. (No cell phones either.)

We had to fight with some of the bystanders until the rescue people came, to keep them from further injuring the victims. For example, one man had been thrown from the car and skidded on his face. Another bystander wanted to turn him over to lie on his back. My husband had to fight with the bystander to keep the man on his side, so he could breathe.

The only person not thrown out of the car was a small baby in a car seat. (This is an argument for seat belts and good infant car seats.) I believe all the people survived, even though they were badly injured.

The Rolled-Over Semi

I took my son and some of his friends to a local amusement park (Valley Fair.) I allowed them to go in together and I stayed in my car to do some work. As I was sitting there, a semi tractor and trailer *slowly* rolled over into the ditch next to the parking lot where I was sitting. It was surreal. I could not believe my eyes. It's hard to believe that a huge truck like that could roll over and especially that it rolled over so slowly. But once a huge truck starts to roll, there is no way to stop it. It seemed like everything was moving in slow motion.

I ran over to see if I could help. The truck driver was pinned in the cab, but he said he didn't think he was badly injured. He was able to call for help on his CB radio. (How I wish we had had cell phones then.) He said he had swerved to miss an oncoming car. (The car did not stop.) There was no way I could get him out of the cab, but I stayed with him until help arrived. The rescue people had to cut him out of the cab, using a tool called "the Jaws of Life," which I had used before.

I asked the driver to call me later and tell me how he was doing. He called and said he was fine. He also said he was very grateful that I was there, because otherwise he would have panicked while he was waiting for help. Again, *a nurse is on duty all the time* and my First Aid training and experience was invaluable.

Upside-Down in the Ditch

When I was enormously pregnant, a car hit me almost head-on. I swerved to try to avoid the crash and ended up in the ditch, with my car lying on the passenger side. The car I was driving was the car that replaced the Volkswagen bug. (Chapter 4) It was *my first car with seat belts*. Since this was in the early days of seat belts (1966), all it had was a lap belt. I did use the seat belt faithfully, even though most people did not have them or did not use them in those days.

The problem was that I was hanging up near the driver's side door in my seat belt, *with the car lying on its other side*. The police had a huge problem trying to figure out how to get me out without dropping me. They couldn't just unhook or cut the seat belt. Finally, they knocked out the windshield and about five guys got under me, to hold me up when they released the seat belt. This took about a half hour to plan and implement.

Then, after they got me out of the car, I walked around for another half hour. Someone finally said, "You should sit down. You might be injured." Nobody thought of it before that. And, neither did I. My First Aid training failed me, because I was probably in shock.

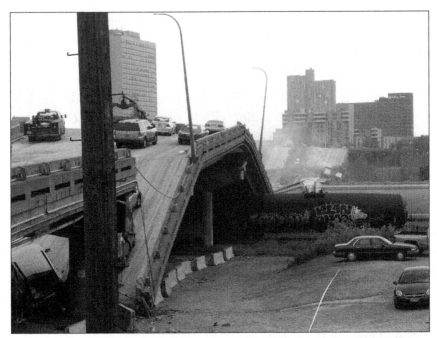

The collapse of the I-35W Mississippi River bridge on August 1, 2007 in Minneapolis left 13 people dead and 145 injured, bringing many emergency patients to local hospitals (Wikimedia)

The man whose car hit me knew it was his fault and was very upset. He was even more upset when he saw that I was very pregnant. He kept in touch with me until after Keith was born, to make sure we were both okay. And, he sent Keith a Baptism gift when the notice was in the local paper. *I believe my Chevy with the seat belts saved my life and that of my son that day. And I am certainly grateful that I was no longer driving the VW bug!*

The Collapse of the Bridge

On August 1, 2007, the Interstate 35W bridge near the University of Minnesota suddenly collapsed during rush hour, killing thirteen people and injuring 145. (MPR News, 2017) I had a meeting at the U that night and I also was invited to a picnic. I chose to go to the picnic. Had I gone to the meeting, I would have been very near or on the bridge when it went down.

At the picnic, we heard that a bridge had collapsed. We just thought it was a small bridge somewhere. Little did we realize the enormity of the disaster. When we found out what had happened, I called the hospital and asked if I should come in to work. By that time, so many nurses and doctors had come to help that they said I didn't need to come, particularly since I worked in Psych and not the Emergency Room.

Since the bridge was over the Mississippi River, victims on the west side of the river were brought to our hospital (HCMC.) The people on the other side were taken to other hospitals. The impact on us in Psych was that we discharged anyone we could, to make room for victims of the collapse.

The 9-11 Terrorist Attack on the Twin Towers

When the Twin Towers in New York collapsed after they were attacked by terrorists (the morning of September 11, 2001), all the trauma hospitals in the U.S. were put on alert. It was expected that our Burn Unit in particular, would receive many victims. Sadly however, very few people who were in the towers when they went down survived. So, we did not get transfers.

I was scheduled to work at three PM the afternoon of the attack. When I went to the hospital in downtown Minneapolis, the city had been totally evacuated. Only rescue people and police were present. It was very weird. When I got to the hospital, it had been totally locked down. Armed guards were at the doors. We had to prove who we were and why we were there, in order to get in.

Being at work that day was *very frustrating*. We had many patients from the Middle East and similar areas. The TV stations showed the images of the planes hitting the towers and the towers collapsing. This was repeated many times throughout the entire day. And, every time this was shown, many of our psych patients clapped and cheered and jumped up and down. They were on the side of the terrorists. It was very frustrating and disappointing to see this. And I had a difficult time keeping my mouth shut.

The 9-11 Fishing Trip

As an aside, on September 11th, my nephew Steve was on a fishing trip in the wilderness above the Arctic Circle. It was the type of trip where a pilot brings you to the site and leaves you there and then returns a week later to pick you up. So, they were there with no radio or other means of communication. When the towers went down, all plane flights in the country were grounded. Therefore, their pilot had no way to come back to pick up the fishermen. And, the fishermen had no communication with the outside world, so they had no idea what had happened.

On the day they were scheduled to leave, Steve and his friends ate the last of their food, packed up their tents and equipment, and waited for the plane. The plane did not arrive. So, they decided maybe they had the wrong day. They reassembled the camp, caught fish for supper, and planned to leave the next day. The next day came and went and still there was no plane. Now, they decided the pilot must have had a heart attack or something and they were on their own. Perhaps no one even knew where they were. And, winter was approaching.

They knew they had to get out of there. So, they packed up their stuff and began to walk. They stumbled upon a small village, *bought a car*, and drove to civilization. They finally found a telephone and learned what had happened. But, it was a very frightening experience. I tried to provide listening and emotional support to the men after they got home.

The House Fire Rescue

One early morning, I was driving to my school in Anoka just before Christmas. It was very cold and dark. Out of the corner of my eye, I thought I saw flames at the corner of a house. Something told me it was not my imagination. I turned around and went back to discover the gas meter on the side of the house shooting up flames like an acetylene torch. It was very loud and seemed to be accelerating.

I ran up and banged on the door and a woman in pajamas stumbled out. She was sleepy and confused. I asked who else was in the house. At first, she wasn't sure. She then remembered that her husband was at work and three of her four children were at school. We ran in and got the fourth child and I put the mother and child in my car to keep warm.

I then ran to a neighbor's home to call for help. (No cell phones then.) By the time the fire department and gas company came, the house was totally engulfed in flames. We could hear cans exploding and walls falling down inside the house. Unfortunately, all the family's belongings and Christmas gifts were destroyed, but the family was okay.

I then learned that the house was new; the family had just moved in. Apparently, the new furnace was not installed correctly. It had exploded and the woman was thrown to the floor. It must have happened just before I got there. The woman probably hit her head and that was why she was confused. I realize that my "nursing mind" kicked in and told me to go back and check on the situation. I know I got the two people out just in the nick of time. Certainly, they would have died in the fire otherwise.

After the situation was under control, I left and went to work. Nobody ever knew who I was. But, *I know I saved two lives that day.*

Quack Doctors

The Chiropractor

While I was in college, I went to a chiropractor in downtown Minneapolis. He was older and he assured me he could diagnose and cure any illness I might have, including cancer. He had a machine with levers and buttons, sound effects, and multi-colored flashing lights. This weird machine was connected to a wand which he passed over my body. This all seemed very strange to me, so I contacted the State Chiropractic Association. They checked this man out and determined that he was a fraud. I believe he lost his license. It was unfortunate, because I am sure some of his patients neglected to check out serious illnesses until it was too late. And there are many competent chiropractors who are impacted by a situation like this. (The program "Pawn

Stars" recently looked at a quack machine like this man had, an "Ellis Micro-Dynameter." (Season 16, Episode 16)

The nursing mentality strikes again.

The Psychologist

While I was going through my divorce, I went to a psychologist two or three times for counseling. He practiced in the lower level of his home. Each time, he tried to convince me that I had a sexual hang-up and would feel much better if I would go to bed with him. I refused to do this and stopped seeing him. (In those days, there were no resources for reporting a harassment situation like this.)

On one of my visits an interesting event solidified my concerns about this man. His wife came home from shopping and had forgotten her house keys. So, she knocked on the door of his office. He yelled, screamed, and swore at her, telling her, "Never interrupt me when I am with a client!" (Of course, that would be a problem if he were making out with the client at the time.)

So again, I notified the licensing authority. When I called them, they told me I could not file a complaint unless I actually went to bed with him (and then, it would just be my word against his.) I was unwilling to do this, so I didn't know what to do.

However, it just happened that this man was also employed as a high school psychologist at the high school where I had been the School Nurse. So, I knew a lot of people there. At Anoka TEC, we had a couple of students who had gone to that high school. And now, one of them was having emotional troubles. She talked to her TEC instructor, who came to ask me what to do. It turned out that this female student had been seeing the same psychologist when she was in high school. He had also been molesting her. (Of course, as a high school student, she was under age.) When questioned, she knew several friends who had the same experience with this psychologist while they were high school students. They said they had been coerced to have sex with this man.

I contacted people I knew at the high school and all the girls were willing to testify against the psychologist. He lost his license. If it hadn't been for these high school girls, he would probably still be in practice. And, if the one girl hadn't gone to Anoka TEC, we never would have heard their story.

Adventures in the "City"

The 9-1-1 Call

One night after work at about midnight, I was driving in downtown Minneapolis and I saw a man lying in the gutter. I stopped next to him and called 9-1-1. I didn't want to get out of the car, in case it was a trap.

The 9-1-1 operator asked if he was drunk and I said I didn't know. I told her I didn't want to get out of the car in the middle of the night.

The operator then asked if the man was Black or White and I said I didn't know, because I didn't want to get out of my car. (From where I was, I actually thought he looked Native American.)

She asked if he was breathing and if he had a pulse. Again, I said I didn't know.

She kept asking questions and I repeated that she should send a police officer, because I was not going to get out of the car in the middle of the night in the middle of the city. I said I would stay there in my car, blocking the man from traffic until the police got there. Finally, an officer came, but I couldn't understand why the 9-1-1 operator kept asking questions and why she didn't understand that it would be dangerous for me to get out of the car. It turned out that the man was inebriated and had just passed out in the street.

Adventures in the "Country"

"I know you're in there."

We lived in an old farm house out in the country. One night, a car followed me home. Like a dummy, I drove into our long, deserted driveway and the car followed me in, blocking my exit. I ran into the house and called my first husband, Ted. He said he couldn't leave the Dairy Queen, which we owned. I should have called the police, but I was scared. So, I grabbed a shotgun and some shells and went upstairs. (*The only phone in the house was downstairs.*)

We had two big black Labrador retriever dogs, so I stationed one by the back door and took one upstairs with me. I sat there like Annie Oakley, wondering if I would ever have the nerve to shoot someone. The guy was walking around the house, talking and banging on the doors. "I know you're in there. Open the door!" I had no idea if he was alone or if someone else was also there, because he was talking. The downstairs dog was barking wildly.

Finally, Ted decided to come home. The guy turned out to be someone he knew. He was drunk and said, "I thought she was my girl friend." Of course, that was ridiculous. He asked if the dog would bite and we said the dog was very vicious. (He had never been aggressive in his life.) Ted refused to press charges. I should have been more assertive. But, I did use my psych nursing skills to talk to this man. He never bothered me again.

The Lady who Collapsed in Church

We moved to a new community and changed churches. Shortly after we moved there, an older lady collapsed in front of me during the service. I went to help her. I had her lying on a pew, with her head lowered, and had someone call 9-1-1.

Suddenly, a woman came up to me, pushed me out of the way, and said, "I am a nurse." I said, "So am I," so then we took care of her together. Nurses always respond when someone needs help. The other nurse didn't know me, so she stepped in to assist. It turned out that I had much more emergency and rescue experience than she did.

The Mountain Rescue

No matter where you are, you are still a nurse and people know it. I was backpacking in the Tetons with my son Keith, who was about ten years old at that time, and several other people.

First, we backpacked up to Jenny Lake and a mountain climbing expedition was to start from there. Several members of our group were going to climb Mount Teewinot. This peak is very difficult and the sixth highest in the Tetons (12,330 feet above sea level), only a few feet shorter than 'the Grand' (13,775 feet.)

Keith said, "I think I could do that. It doesn't look too hard." And I said, "Absolutely not!" (I stayed at the bottom of the mountain with Keith.)

The group successfully climbed the peak, but then snow conditions changed. The climbers did not put on crampons and one of the men (Harold) slipped. His son (Danny) tried to grab him, but was unsuccessful. Harold slid to the bottom of the couloir (steep passage or gully) and landed on the rocks, hitting his head. Danny fell into a crevasse (crevice or fissure) and was trapped.

I thought I heard a faint "Caroline" several times and finally realized it really was someone calling me. Members of the group were calling for help from the mountaintop. When I got to the bottom of the mountain, Harold was unconscious, but his pulse and respiration were okay. I stopped the bleeding in his head wound as much as I could, and covered him up.

The Portland Climbing Club was also on the mountain and they had managed to notify the Rangers of the accident. This club was working to extricate Danny from the crevasse. The Rangers arrived very quickly. (They came straight up the mountainside, not on the trail.) Two of them were carrying a metal basket stretcher, each having half on their back. They, of course, had First Aid equipment.

When I reported Harold's vital signs, the Rangers handed me a walkie-talkie and said, "Here. Push this button to talk." They then continued up to assist in extricating Danny. It turned out that I was talking to the Emergency Room at the Jackson Hole, Wyoming hospital. I gave them all the details and they sent a helicopter to transport Harold.

After Danny was pulled out of the crevasse, he was brought down by the Climbing Club and the Rangers. A second helicopter was sent to transport him to the hospital. Suddenly, we realized that all the gear (including tents, backpacks, and boots) for the two injured men was still on the mountain. We had absolutely no way to carry it all down.

So, we had to quickly pack up their stuff and a third helicopter was sent to pick up this equipment.

After the third helicopter left, Keith quietly said, "*Maybe it's harder than it looks!*"

By this time, it was too late to hike out, so we had to stay overnight. We had no idea how the men were doing. Danny's fiancé, Lisa, was very worried. The next day when we got off the mountain, we found the two men sitting on a park bench in front of the hospital without boots (which had been removed by the Rangers.) They were doing okay, except the father had had a concussion.

Once a nurse, always a nurse! All the time. Everywhere.

Weight-Loss Surgery

Weight-loss (*bariatric*) surgery has been performed for nearly fifty years. It had begun at hospitals such as the University of Minnesota during my student days. (Chapter 2) However, in the past twenty-plus years, laparoscopic procedures (through a tiny wound) have made it much safer and more comfortable for the patient. It has been estimated that by 2011, 340,000 laparoscopic bariatric procedures had been performed worldwide. (Wikipedia, 2018)

One morbidly obese patient MaryJane had recently remarried. She was approaching forty and desperately wanted to have a child. She had weight-loss surgery and lost a great deal of weight. She got pregnant and had a daughter. Then, she began overeating and gradually stretched her stomach out again. She has now regained all the weight lost, plus more. But, she does have a wonderful daughter. (Only about five percent of morbidly obese people maintain their large weight loss after surgery.)

Another patient had weight-loss surgery and lost more than 100 pounds. She then worked for a weight loss program. They showed "before" and "after" photos of her and gave the impression that she had lost the weight there, rather than as a result of her surgery. However, she has kept the weight off. (Another patient said she couldn't believe how much more water it took to fill the bathtub after she lost over 100 pounds!)

Property Management—Preparation for Psychiatry

Over the years, my second husband Ron and I had a number of rental properties. It seemed that Ron always sent me to take care of problems in these units. Sometimes, psych experience comes in handy.

The Gang Members

One property was in Delano, Minnesota. Every time I called, a different person answered the phone. So, I could not figure out who was actually living there. When I checked, I learned that an entire motorcycle gang was living in the tiny two-bedroom house.

So, I went out *alone* to meet with the tenants and tell them they had to move out. We were out in the back yard and I was surrounded by about eight motorcycle guys. They were smoking cigarettes and pulling knives out of their boots to open beer bottles. It really never occurred to me to be scared, but I probably should have been. I talked to them respectfully and explained that the house was too small for all of them and they moved out without incident.

Later, it dawned on me that they could have killed me and I would not have been able to defend myself against all of them. But, it was good that I had psych experience and had worked with all types of people. (And, why did I go out there alone?)

The "Poor Farm"

Another property was the former Wright County "Poor Farm" just north of Buffalo, Minnesota. There were six little apartments there. One night, we got a call from the Sheriff saying that a group of our tenants had robbed a local restaurant and bar and had gone back to our apartment building.

The Sheriff asked me to go out to the place with him, because he wasn't sure what would happen. (He always asked me to go with him if he thought my nursing experience would help.) Since these men were our tenants, he figured I would know how to deal with them. He may have even been afraid of them. I had no idea what we would find—maybe drugs; maybe guns . . .

When we got there, one of the guys was the son of a friend of mine. He was pretty surprised and embarrassed to see me and vice versa. They surrendered the liquor and money they had stolen. I think they got off with just probation, but I am not sure. My mental health nursing skills came in very handy that night.

Bats in the "Belfry"

We also had an infestation of bats at the Poor Farm. It was a large and very old building with an open, unoccupied attic. Occasionally, the bats from the attic ventured out into the apartments. Obviously, the tenants were afraid of them. And bats can carry various diseases, including rabies. So, we knew we had to get rid of them. We called several exterminators before we could find one who wanted to deal with bats.

We learned that bats are very difficult to keep out, once they have established a home. I know bats eat pests, such as mosquitoes, but you don't want them in your home. (We had to catch a couple of them and have them tested for diseases by the State Health Department. That was an exciting adventure.)

The exterminators had to first get every bat out of the attic (at the same time.) They then had to fill any TINY hole, because bats can get through very tiny openings (much smaller than half a dime.) Bats will always try to return to their original home.

It was a long and expensive project, but we did eradicate the bats. So, we did not have any more "bats in the belfry." And thankfully, nobody got sick or attacked by the bats.

The Old Lady and the Judge

The lower level of our duplex in Waverly, Minnesota was occupied by a little old lady. For a few months, she decided she didn't have to pay rent. We disagreed and tried to evict her. I tried to talk to her, to no avail.

She sued us for harassment, so we had to go to court. The judge was also an older man and he knew her. He took her side. He said it was terrible that we were treating an elderly lady that way and ruled in her favor, even though she was clearly wrong.

She did move out, but we never got our money. (Small-town court—EEK.) My psychiatric skills did not work with that lady or with the judge.

The Man on the Bandstand

We also had a duplex in Dassel, Minnesota. The upstairs was occupied by a man who was clearly psychotic. Each month, I had to go out there to collect the rent, but he always paid. Sometimes, his mind was together; sometimes, he was clearly responding to internal stimuli (hearing voices, *hallucinations*.) I liked him and we would have "counseling sessions." I was kind of like his monthly Public Health Nurse.

Usually, when he was displaying symptoms, he would admit he was off his meds. Then, I would encourage him to start taking them again. If he couldn't pay for them, I would arrange for the county to pay for them. Then, he would get better for a while.

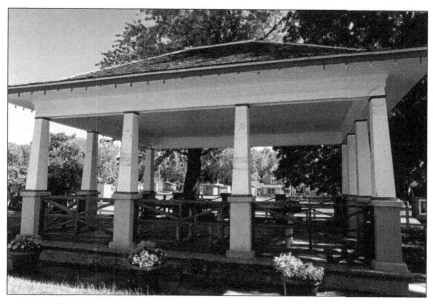

Rosdahl collected rent from a Dassel resident who was sitting on top of the bandstand, as his monthly "public health psych nurse" (CB Rosdahl)

One day, I banged on his door and got no answer. The neighbor lady came out and silently just pointed to the park across the street. I looked up and there he was, *on top of the bandstand!* So, here I was, out in the park looking up at this man on top of the bandstand, telling him he had to pay his rent. It had to have been a funny picture. And, he climbed down and paid his rent. (This was also good preparation for later working in the Mental Health Unit at HCMC.)

Four Fractures, an Infection, and a T. and A.

The Bicycle Accident

When I was about nine years old, I was riding my bike on the highway. I didn't look and was hit by a car. I skidded on the highway and, since I was wearing only my bathing suit, most of the skin on my body was scraped off.

The man who hit me stopped and was very kind. I asked him if he would "please carry my bike home." I walked in the door of my house and my parents nearly fainted. They had me lie down on the couch. After lying down, I could not move.

There was almost no ambulance service in those days, so my father picked me up and put me in the car. When we got to the doctor's office (which was upstairs), my father carried me up. Then, several people held me down and they put mercurochrome all over my body. So, now I was orange.

I had a fractured pelvis. I was so fortunate that I did not have a spinal injury or I would have been paralyzed for sure. Today, after that accident, I would have had a cervical collar and would have been strapped to a backboard before being transported. (Good training for rescue missions in the future.)

The Golf Course Accident

I was playing golf with my son, husband, and daughter-in-law Kim, (who is a nurse.) I started sliding down a small slippery hill. I figured if I sat down, I would not get hurt. However, my foot got caught and I sat on my ankle. I knew it was fractured. Kim asked if I was okay and I said "no." Typical nurse, she said, "*Yes, I heard it snap.*"

I didn't want to disrupt everyone's game, particularly since it was my son's birthday, so I said I would wait in the car. They got me some ice and I had to sit there in silence until they came back.

We went to the Emergency Room and they said, "We will put you in the hospital and do surgery in the morning." I had not had dinner yet, so I insisted that they put on a splint and I would come back in the morning. Typical nurse. (They said they knew I was a nurse, because I rated my pain at a "two, out of ten!")

The surgery consisted of the insertion of pins and rods, held in place with screws. It was done with spinal anesthesia, so I was able to watch the whole procedure, because I was awake. It was the strangest sensation to see my leg lifted up. I knew it was my leg, but I couldn't feel anything. I have lumps in my ankle where the screws are and one of the screws has worked out a little bit. My husband says I "have a screw loose." And now I can predict changes in the weather, as indicated by pain.

The Iowa Tumble

Recently, we were at an event in Iowa and I tripped on the sidewalk. I skidded on my face and hands and even skinned my toes (because I was wearing sandals). I looked like I had been attacked. We went to a local ER and they splinted my wrist and told me to see my own doctor to see if it was fractured. (*Of course, they took me aside and asked me several times if I was being abused by anyone, because I was so beat up.* They were more concerned about that than they were about my wrist injury.)

When I went to my own doctor, he said I should see an Orthopedic specialist. I asked if my wrist was fractured, and he said he wasn't

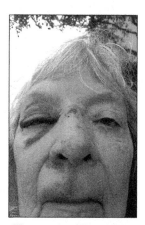

The result of Rosdahl's fall in Iowa—medical people couldn't believe she wasn't being abused at home
(BH Media)

177

sure. (People at that doctor's office also asked if I was being abused by someone.)

So, next I went to the Orthopedist. I asked if my wrist was fractured and he said, "Of course it is—in three places!" I don't know why nobody else would tell me. The next words out of his mouth were, "Now, at your age, you can choose whether or not to have surgery."

He then went on to say, "If you were any older, I wouldn't give you a choice." I wanted to talk to him about his choice of words, but I controlled myself. (I know I am old, but he didn't have to point it out.) I chose not to have surgery, so I have a deformed wrist, but it works just fine.

The Small Town Hospital

We were in a small town north of Minneapolis, helping our son, Keith, to move. My husband, Ron, fell off the truck and broke his wrist in several places. I splinted it tightly with magazines and we went to the local small town hospital for treatment. Since it was Sunday, the "doctor" on call was very young. I am not sure if he was actually a licensed MD or if he was still in school.

Ron's arm was crooked, as the bones were overlapped. The "doctor" didn't have a clue as to what to do. So, I took him out in the hall and told him what I thought would work. I told him to fasten Ron's hand up, hanging from an IV pole. Then, he could pull down on Ron's elbow and the bones should snap back into place. He said, "Do you think that would work?" and I said that it should.

So, the doctor went back into the room and said, *"I have decided . . ."* and went on to tell Ron what I had told him. He did what I said to do and the bones snapped back into place. And the "doctor" said, "Well, I'll be damned!" (He probably used that technique again in his medical practice and never told anyone how he learned to do it.)

As always, the nurse is constantly on duty. Ron still needed surgery, but was able to wait until he could see his own doctor after the weekend.

The Infection

I had major surgery and then went to Arkansas (too soon.) It was a holiday weekend (probably Christmas) and everyone was going on vacation. I got a terrible infection. I was running a very high fever (103-104 degrees F.) and was in a *huge amount of pain* (**ten plus.**) I had taken so many painkillers that I was afraid the doctor would accuse me of overdosing.

Because we were not home, I did not have a doctor in Arkansas. I was told on the phone by my doctor in Minnesota that I had to see a specialist and not a General Practitioner. So, I called a specialist's office in Hot Springs. I was told that I could not be seen for four days. *After the holiday weekend.*

I knew (being a nurse) that the infection was so bad that I needed to be seen *immediately.* I tried to explain this to the person who answered the phone and she did not care. She would not give me an appointment. I was becoming desperate. I knew that if I waited four days, I might not live.

So, I called the local hospital Emergency Room and asked what doctor was on call for that particular specialty. They told me and I called that doctor's office. I was told the same thing—I could not be seen until after the holiday week end.

So, I said, "I cannot wait. I am critically ill. Let me tell you what I am going to do. I will wait until about six or seven o'clock this evening and then I will go to the Emergency Room at the hospital. Then your doctor on-call will have to come and see me. OR, you can give me an appointment earlier today and we can get this resolved." She consulted with someone and *suddenly they had an available appointment.*

When I saw the doctor, he told me that he would start me on a massive dose of oral antibiotics. If I was not better by evening, I was to come to the hospital, where I would be admitted and would receive IV antibiotics. He said if I had waited four days, *I would probably not have survived*, which I knew. (I told him how I had gotten the appointment. I hope he talked to his receptionist.)

The antibiotics did the trick and I was okay. But, if I had not been a nurse, I would probably have waited and may have died. Sometimes, you just have to use your nursing judgment and advocate for yourself.

The T. and A.

When I was very young, I needed to have my tonsils and adenoids removed. (Called a "T. & A.") I did not want to be "put to sleep," so they agreed to do it with Novocaine. (I was much too young to make that decision.) I was placed in a *dental chair* and Novocain was injected into the back of my throat.

This was the worst decision of my life and I still gag very easily. They should not have allowed me to make the decision not to have general anesthesia. As a nurse, I have advised other parents not to allow a very young child to have local anesthesia for this procedure.

A Special Trip

The Launch of the Space Shuttle

Because I was a nurse and a school administrator, my husband Ron and I were invited by NASA and the US Navy to be guests at a special trip to observe a launch of the Space Shuttle in Florida. NASA said they particularly wanted me to come, because I was a nurse and also because I had had experience with the Hyperbaric Chamber.

We traveled by bus from Minnesota with a group of other teachers and administrators. We were treated royally and several

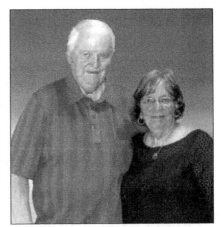

Caroline Rosdahl and husband, Ron Christensen, while on a trip (BH Media)

tours were conducted for us. We toured the Space Center and the huge aircraft carrier, the Roosevelt. It was hard to believe how enormous the ship was.

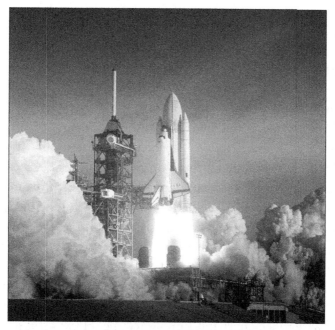

Viewing the launch of the Space Shuttle in Florida was a
special trip for educators (Wikimedia)

At Cape Canaveral for the launch, we were seated on special bleachers. They were located as close to the launch as allowed for civilians. Many other spectators were camped out on the beaches and parked on all roads surrounding the Cape.

From our vantage point, we could hear the countdown. When the Shuttle launched, we could feel the ground shake and feel the heat from the blast. It was an amazing experience. And, I remembered the visit with General Taylor at the Pentagon in 1958, when he showed us the movie of the first satellite. (Chapter 2)

Now, we were seeing it in person.

After the launch, we were bused to Huntsville, Alabama, to see the underwater training areas for the astronauts. These facilities are used to assist the astronauts to deal with weightlessness, among other things. It reminded me of my work in the Hyperbaric Chamber at Minneapolis General Hospital. (Chapter 5) And, I understood some of the problems with diving and decompression (from my hyperbaric chamber time.) I was able to explain some of this to the other guests.

FAMILY STORIES AND OTHER TRIVIA

The Prospective Tracheostomy

When I was a nursing student, I was in the University Hospital, where I had a severe allergic reaction. An intern enthusiastically approached my bed with a "trach" tray. I told him that as long as I was conscious, he was not allowed to "practice" on me. (A "trach" involves an opening in the patient's throat, to facilitate breathing.) He was disappointed, because when they gave me emergency epinephrine and it worked, I was able to breathe. So he didn't get to practice his trach skills that day!

"My IV Froze!"

Years later, I was in the hospital in midwinter. It was about twenty degrees below zero. My husband Ron visited me. He was still smoking at the time, so he went outside to have a cigarette. He met a lady outside in her hospital gown and bathrobe in the bitter cold. He said, "This must be miserable for you to have to go out in this cold." She replied, "Yes, but yesterday was worse. My IV froze." (I would imagine it would be hazardous to your health to have *ice-cold fluid flowing into your vein.*)

Pneumonia

An older relative of Ron's was in the hospital. He was very ill and was in the ICU. When we went to visit him, he had been moved out of ICU into a regular Medicine Unit. I listened to him breathe and I said, "He has pneumonia." I talked to his nurse and she said, "Oh, he just got out of ICU. He will be okay."

I did not believe he would be okay, so I demanded to see the doctor. As soon as the doctor saw him he said, "He has pneumonia. He needs to go back into the ICU." I had been correct about his condition. He was returned to the ICU and we felt comfortable enough to go home.

However, back in the ICU, a nurse gave him a cardiac medication by the wrong route. It was supposed to be given into his NG (nasogastric) tube, which was in his stomach. She gave it IV, directly into the vein. This was too much for his system and he died almost immediately. I felt very badly, because if I had been there I may have been able to prevent the error.

The hospital did call us and admit their mistake, but it was heartbreaking. Nurses have the patients' lives in their hands.

Keith's Medical Adventures

The Arkansas Dentist

We had a vacation home in Arkansas. Once, when we were down there from Minnesota, I broke a tooth, so I had to find a dentist. I just picked someone at random from the phone book. He turned out to be an older man and was very kind. I liked him, so my husband and I both went to him several times.

One time, I had just gotten photos that were taken when my twin grand-daughters, Emily and Bailey, were at the dentist. They were about two or three-years-old at the time. I was looking at the photos while waiting to see the dentist. The receptionist said, "It looks like the children were at the dentist." And I said that was true. She asked if they could have prints of these photos to put up in their office, to encourage people to bring in their young children. So, I made prints for her.

Shortly after that, my husband went to this same dentist. He came home and said, "They have photos of two kids in there and they look just like Emily and Bailey." I had to laugh because he didn't realize that the photos WERE Emily and Bailey.

Keith's Stay at Mercy Hospital

When my son, Keith, was about a year and a half old, we were afraid he might have cystic fibrosis. He was hospitalized at Mercy Hospital, where my PN students from Anoka were having their hands-on clinical experience. So, they all paid a lot of attention to him. Keith was very rambunctious and an excellent jumper. The staff was afraid he would

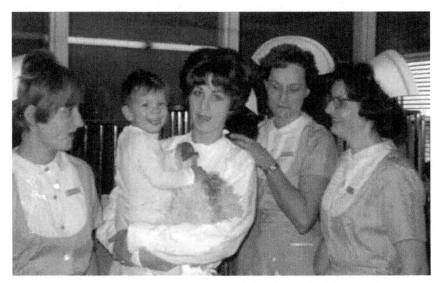

Rosdahl's son, Keith, as a patient in Mercy Hospital, 1968—Anoka TEC PN students gave him very special attention (CB Rosdahl)

jump out of the crib, so they had to put a net over the top of the crib. (And as it turned out, thank goodness, he did not have any serious illness.)

The Scary Babysitter

Early in my career at Anoka, I took Keith to the home of a babysitter in the Anoka area. She was an older lady and seemed very devoted to Keith. One day, I had an evening meeting, so I arranged for one of my students (Sharon), to pick up Keith. I told the lady ahead of time and she said that was fine.

Later, I got a call from Sharon and she said the babysitter had refused to let her take Keith. The babysitter had said to her, "*You can't have him. He's my baby.*" Of course, I immediately went over and picked him up. I had him safely in my car with Sharon and then I went back in and told the babysitter he would not be coming back. Ever. I was really frightened that she was planning to kidnap him.

Twenty-Three Buttons

Right after the preceding incident, I began having Keith stay near my home with a friend, Patty. One day I went to pick him up and Patty said, "I have been finding Keith with buttons all day. I have taken them away from him, but I didn't know where he was getting them. I don't think he has put any in his mouth." (Ho, ho, ho; right?) She said, "I finally discovered that my button bag had fallen off the closet shelf and Keith was picking things out from under the door with his tiny fingers."

My major concern was that there were also pins and needles in the button bag. I could not believe he had not swallowed any of the buttons or other stuff. So, I immediately took him to the ER. (Nurse's instinct.)

At the hospital, they took an x-ray, which showed *twenty-three buttons, throughout his entire digestive tract*. He had been putting them in his mouth, and of course, swallowing them, all day. There were no pins or needles. So, it was no big deal, but it was a very funny x-ray. (I wish I had a copy of it now.)

The Soccer Injury

Keith decided to play soccer when he was about eight. The very first day, someone stepped on his finger. The playground was right next to the hospital, so Keith took himself over to the E.R. and said he wanted to be treated. They asked where his parents were and he said he had just brought himself. He is a nurse's son, after all. Of course, we had to come and sign him in, but he was resourceful. He gave up soccer that very day.

Ron's Medical Adventures

The Confusing Hospital Stay

In 2017, we drove pretty much straight through from Minneapolis to Allentown, Pennsylvania for a car show. On the last evening, we went to an awards dinner. During the dinner, Ron began to have chest pains and was having trouble breathing. They had paramedics at the dinner, so I asked them to check him out. They put him on a rolling gurney and had ECG (electrocardiogram) patches all over his body. They were also giving him oxygen. I didn't think it was his heart, but was not sure.

Just as all this was going on, the dinner was over. All the people from home were asking what was going on and how Ron was doing. There was such a big crowd, the rescuers had trouble getting through. Finally, they got him loaded into an ambulance. Ron was taken (by ambulance) to an Urgent Care *across the street*. They decided they couldn't handle the situation there, so he was loaded back into the ambulance for a trip to a regular hospital. The ambulance people asked if I wanted to ride along, but I said "no," because I needed to have a car available.

We were in a strange city and I had no idea where they were going. The ambulance people told me how to get there and it was very confusing. So, I told them I was going to follow them and to be sure not to lose me. As it turned out, they did not go the way they had told me, so I would have been really lost.

When we got to the hospital, Ron was admitted and it was determined that he had built up blood clots in his legs (*thrombophlebitis*) during the long drive. These clots now became *emboli* in both his lungs. This can be a very life-threatening situation, but Ron was doing pretty well.

On admission to his hospital room, two doctors were at his bedside *arguing about what to do*. Ron, the patient, and I were right there. They were arguing about what kind of IV to give him. I suggested that they go out in the hall to decide what to do.

They finally started an IV and gave him some medications. I gave them a list of the medications he was taking at home and they ordered *only some of them*. There were some medications that they didn't even have at that hospital, so I had to go to a drug store and get them myself.

One day, a nursing assistant was trying to take a blood sample. She obviously didn't know what she was doing, so she stuck him several times. And, she spilled blood on the floor, *which remained there for about twenty-four hours*.

Ron was in the hospital for three days and *they never offered him a backrub, comb, toothbrush, or washcloth.* Not even after he went to the bathroom or before he ate! He was supposed to walk, but I had to accompany him, because they never did. His roommate was an elderly, confused man. He kept trying to get out of bed, setting off an alarm, so Ron couldn't get any sleep.

Finally, I demanded that they figure out what medications he should have, so I could take him home to Minnesota. One medication was ordered as *four tablets twice a day.* They gave him a prescription for ten tablets total. This might get us to Ohio! I had to talk to the chief of the department to get an appropriate prescription.

When we got back to Minnesota, we got a questionnaire asking about his care. I could not help myself. I filed a complaint (which I have NEVER done before.) Then, I got a call from the head nurse (who had some other fancy title.) I was trying to be nice, so I said, "I understand that you might have been short-staffed." And, she exclaimed, "Oh no. We were fully staffed." I could not believe what she said. Again, I simply could not help myself and I said, "Then, that makes it even worse." She then realized that what she had said sounded really dumb.

Later, I was telling a friend about all this and she said, "Well, Southern hospitals may have problems." I pointed out that Pennsylvania is NOT Southern. All in all, it was an interesting and frightening experience. I can't imagine what would have happened to Ron if I had not been a nurse. I could at least take care of some of the details. And, I certainly would not ever go back to that hospital.

The Stroke

I came home one very hot summer day and Ron was lying on the couch, which he never did during the day. He had been playing golf all day and drinking only Diet Pepsi. He was obviously dehydrated. When I asked him what was going on, he said, "salkxnssognlknallg." He was mumbling for sure. I told him I was going to call the ambulance and he said, "No, dlckhsoslalnglaglsal." The only word I could understand was "no," which being a nurse, I ignored.

Of course, I did call the ambulance. When he got to the hospital, they determined that he had had a heat stroke, but to me it looked exactly like a CVA (cerebral vascular accident—stroke.) Given fluids and electrolytes, he was just fine. I do hope he learned something about outdoor activities in extreme heat. And I learned about a regular stroke versus heat-related problems.

Shoveling the Sidewalk

One very snowy evening, Ron had a very bad cold. He was so weak; he couldn't get out of his recliner chair. I suggested he get on his hands and knees and maybe he could pull himself up. This was worse. He is much too heavy for me to lift. So, I finally called 9-1-1 for help. Apparently, they get many similar calls for help.

The police arrived and then the fire truck. The firemen came in and had Ron off the floor and into bed within minutes. Then, one of the firemen asked, "Where is your shovel? You haven't shoveled your sidewalk." So, he got the shovel and cleaned the snow off the sidewalk. This was so nice and I was really impressed. What kind men they were! So, I guess if you are a rescue person, there are unplanned duties as well.

Two Nosebleed (*Epistaxis*) Stories

A Nosebleed at the Hospital

One day when I was working at HCMC, I got a very severe nosebleed. The nurses and Nurse Practitioner were unable to stop the bleeding, so I was taken to the Emergency Room. When I got there, I was taken *immediately* into a Treatment Room. The doctor came in right away. He cauterized my nose and placed a packing. The bleeding was stopped.

I expressed my thanks and told him I was very grateful to have been seen so quickly, since the waiting room was full of patients waiting to be seen. He said, "Oh, that's nothing. We just didn't want you to bleed all over the floor in the waiting room!"

The "Fatal" Nosebleed

It was Christmas Eve and I was scheduled to read the Scripture at the midnight church service. About ten PM, I got an arterial nosebleed. It was gushing all over and I couldn't get it stopped. I decided I should go to the Emergency Room at the nearest community hospital by ambulance, since it would take about twenty minutes to get there. I didn't want to bleed all over our car and I didn't want Ron to have to take care of me and also drive. And, in case I passed out, the EMTs could take care of me. So, we called the ambulance and asked for transport—no lights and siren.

Ron drove separately (and actually beat the ambulance to the hospital.) I was riding in the ambulance and I told the EMT I needed to call my pastor. She said, "Well, we will get you to the hospital soon and then you can call."

And, we drove on, driving slowly in towns and on the highway. After about ten more minutes, I said, "I really need to call my pastor NOW." And the EMT said, "You're going to be OK, honey."

This struck me funny. I realized she believed that I thought I might die on the way to the hospital with a nosebleed. When I explained the situation to her, we got a good laugh.

CHAPTER 9

TEACHING EXPERIENCES

In addition to teaching in the Practical Nursing Program in Anoka, and teaching First Aid and the Nursing Assistant students at Hopkins, I have also taught at every other level of nursing. Most of my teaching positions have been part-time, while I had other full-time employment. Had I not had a Baccalaureate Degree in Nursing, I would not have been eligible to teach most of these classes.

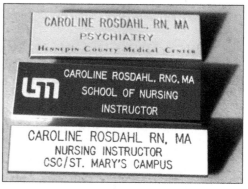

Name badges from part-time teaching positions (CB Rosdahl)

Any nurse who plans to teach will often have adventures that are different than those experienced in the hospital. And, I taught at some unusual locations, considering my nursing background.

- While in graduate school, I was the Evening Clinical Instructor for the three-year-diploma nursing program at Northwestern Hospital.

- While at the Eye Bank, I taught basic nursing classes, part-time, in the St. Mary's Junior College two-year RN program, now a part of St. Catherine's University.

191

- While at Hennepin County Medical Center, I taught Community Psych in the U of Minnesota four-year BSN degree program.

- For over twenty years, I taught in the Department of Vocational-Technical Education at the U. These were courses required for state Licensure as a Vo-Tech teacher. (I believe Marilyn and I were the only nurses and the only females who ever taught any of these classes. (Chapter 6)

- I also supervised Vocational-Technical Education student teachers from St. Cloud State University. It was very unusual for a nurse to be in this position.

Be flexible.
I particularly like a saying I have seen. I do not know the source. *"A school is four walls with tomorrow inside."*

Northwestern Hospital School of Nursing
I worked only evenings, so I was the only instructor in the hospital after about five PM. Anything that came up was my responsibility. The students often invited me to eat with them. When the Program Director found out, she called me in. She said it was "very unprofessional" for me to be "fraternizing with the students." So, I usually ate alone.

When is Your Baby Due?
On my first day of teaching there, I was very pregnant. I went to lunch with some other instructors during the day. I had spaghetti and meatballs and dropped a meatball. It bounced about four times down my big stomach on my brand new white uniform. Great way to make an impression when meeting new people! I had my baby early, very shortly after I started the job at Northwestern. I went back soon after Keith's birth, so I was still carrying some "baby weight."

One of the students said, "You must be our new Instructor" and introduced herself. Then she asked, "When is your baby due?" I had to tell her I had already had him. She was very embarrassed and I felt sorry for her.

The New Nursing Graduate

I was supposed to team-teach some lectures with a new baccalaureate RN graduate from a small college in Southern Minnesota. One day, she was teaching how to empty a catheter bag. In those days, you had to use sterile technique to disconnect the catheter tubing, in order to empty the collection bag.

She did not keep the ends sterile when she did the demonstration. So after class, very nicely, I tried to explain to her the prevention of bladder infections, by keeping the ends of the tubing sterile. She became very angry and said I didn't know what I was talking about and, furthermore, "It was none of my business." So, I taught my own classes and refused to attend hers. I think she left before the year was over. I never saw her again after the day of the catheter class.

Clinical Stories: Checking CMS

One day, a young female student was assigned to a young man about her age. He had a fractured leg. His leg was in a full cast. I asked her to check his CMS (color, motion, and sensitivity.) This involves checking the patient's foot and toes, to make sure the circulation is intact. The student came back to me and said, "The color looks fine, it moves easily, and he wasn't even too embarrassed." I asked her, with fear and trepidation, what she had checked—*and it wasn't his toes!* I would like to have seen his face and gritted teeth during this penis exam.

The Intercom

Another evening, I told a student to check with four-year-old Bobby on the Intercom, to see if he needed anything. She pushed the intercom button and said, "Bobby." No answer. She repeated this, again with no answer.

The third time, she said, "Bobby!" louder. And, a tiny little scared voice said, "What do you want, Wall?" I suggested she go in and teach Bobby how to use the intercom.

Students of Note

Hubert Humphrey's daughter was one of our students. (Humphrey [1911-1978] was a very important Minnesotan. He was mayor of Minneapolis from 1945-1948, U.S. Senator representing Minnesota from 1949-1964, and again from 1971-1978, and 38th Vice President of the United States from 1965-1969.) Humphrey came to the school occasionally to visit his daughter.

I also had a woman student whose last name was Yarns. As a co-incidence, I later had her husband as a student in the PN program in Anoka. (Chapter 7)

St. Mary's Junior College

I taught students who were in the beginning quarters of their two-year nursing program at St. Mary's. This involved teaching basic nursing procedures—bedmaking, giving bed baths and back rubs, and taking temperature, pulse, respiration, and blood pressure.

It was fun to "get back to my roots." It is amazing how much students learn in a short time. The instructor must remember that fact when teaching beginning students. They need to start from the *very beginning and build upon that*. The instructor needs to *assume they have no background* when they start.

One evening while teaching, I had pain in my side. It was pretty bad, but I decided to wait until my shift was over before going to the ER. When I got to the ER, they found that I had passed a *very large kidney stone*. They were amazed at the size of it and the fact that I kept working. Nurses need to be tough. Never give up!

University of Minnesota School of Nursing

For the U of M School of Nursing, I taught Community Psychiatry. It was a wonderful adjunct to my current work with patients in the Inpatient Psychiatry Unit at HCMC. I supervised students in various community psych-related placements and taught some lecture classes.

Group Homes and Drop-In Centers

One group home was *Bristol Place*, several houses making up a group home campus, near downtown Minneapolis. This was a nice facility, with lots of activities for clients. Barb, one of the staff there, later worked with me at HCMC as a social worker.

Other facilities where our students had clinical experience included *Anchor House*, a group home for women. Here, clients had assignments and helped with cooking and housekeeping. This helped them learn valuable and practical life skills.

Bright Lights on Broadway was a drop-in center. Here, clients socialized and participated in many activities in the community. There were parties, tours, and other social activities. They could also just come to the center and play games or watch TV with other clients. Clients also received assistance for their futures, such as resume' writing, interviewing skills, and housing assistance. Some people were also referred to specific jobs.

Both Anchor House and Bright Lights were in North Minneapolis and I had been told that this could be a dangerous area.

One day, I had to drive our huge vintage 1974 Cadillac convertible to clinical, because my car was in the shop. As I drove through the streets, men on the corners yelled at me—"Bitchin' car, Mama!" and "When can I ride with you?" and "I'm available for adoption." I never had any trouble in that area, however.

People Inc

I also took students to *People Inc* in Northeast Minneapolis. One day, one of my students just decided not to visit her assigned client that day. She did not notify me, the client, or the facility. She and I were called in to meet with the Director of the facility.

The Director told her that if she were employed there, she would have been fired. The girl was unconcerned. When I talked to the on-campus program coordinator, I was told that I couldn't give her a bad grade, because she was Class President and she was due to graduate in a few months. (Th*at would not happen with today's faculty!*)

Harbor Lights

One of the most interesting community placements was Harbor Lights, a large Salvation Army facility near Target Field in downtown Minneapolis. I would never have had occasion to go there had I not been taking nursing students. The services offered to clients, most of whom are homeless, are very impressive. These include a health care clinic and a dental clinic, as well as health counseling and mental health services.

There is a chapel service every evening. And they also serve a full dinner to all comers each evening. The dinner is a balanced meal, including milk, salad, fruits and vegetables. (At one time, they had a van that went around to homeless camps with food. However, this service had to be discontinued. It became too dangerous for the staff, because of drug use in the camps.)

Harbor Lights has showers, washers, and dryers for clients to use. They also have a policy that the "hallways are an extension of the street" in bad weather. When it is very cold, for example, homeless people can sit in the halls or the chapel, to avoid frostbite.

The facility has a designated unit for people with mental health concerns. This was where my students spent the most time. In addition to groups and individual mental health counseling, medications are also available to clients there. Harbor Lights is an excellent example of community Public Health Nursing. It was a great experience for my students (and for me.)

The Beacon Program

The Beacon Program at Harbor Lights serves chemically dependent men from all over the U.S. One requirement for admission is having previously failed in several other treatment facilities. (The Beacon Program has about the same success rate as many well-known CD treatment centers.)

One day, I was sitting in on a group and a huge, tall man had on fuzzy duck slippers, with large formed ducks' heads on the toes. They were about size fourteen. I couldn't stop looking at these slippers, because they looked so out of place. He noticed this and told me his sister had given them to him for good luck. He had a good sense of humor about it.

The Beacon Program also assists clients to find employment and allows them to live at Harbor Lights for a time until they can manage on their own. In addition to being safe, this is an advantage for them, because they have an address and phone number where prospective employers can contact them.

Help with Housing

One problem facing homeless people, particularly those who are mentally ill, is housing. In the past, there were many SROs (*Single Room Occupancy* units) available, but many of these have been torn down to make way for condos. Harbor Lights had a few small apartments, but more recently, they have built Hope Harbor. This is a large ninety-six-unit building across the street from the main facility. Here, clients can live, paying affordable rent, as long as they maintain the expectations of the community. (For example: no drugs, no guns.) Rent assistance is also available to many clients at Hope Harbor.

U of M Vocational Education Department

Team-teaching the first Voc-Ed course that Marilyn Cheney and I taught was limited by the Voc-Ed Department to health occupations teachers only. (Chapter 6) The "higher-ups" did not think we "girls" could teach people like Auto Mechanics, Welders, or Electricians.

The next course we taught, we were assigned to "team-teach" with a long-time Vo-Tech male teacher. This was pretty funny, because Marilyn and I had objectives and course outlines and everything was organized. However, on the days this man was supposed to teach, it was totally different. He would come into the classroom, sit on the desk, and say, "Okay. What do you people want to talk about today?"

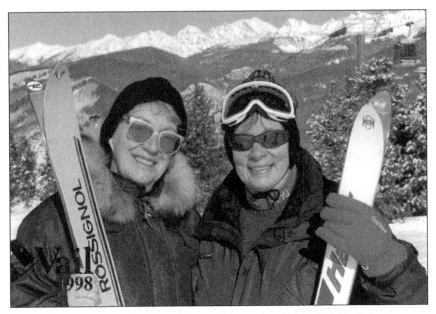

Rosdahl with Marilyn Cheney Stern on a ski trip (BH Media)

Marilyn and I had to prove ourselves, since the department had never had female teachers or nurses before. Gradually, we gained credibility. We taught and I taught alone. Eventually, we were teaching required courses for all Vocational Education teachers. The U finally decided that women could successfully teach people other than nurses, even if the students were men. Teaching is teaching, no matter who the students are. (Marilyn completed her PhD, married, and moved away.) After she left, I continued teaching courses in the Department for a number of years.

Marilyn and I remained friends and even went sailing and skiing together.

The Itinerant Teacher
I taught Voc-Ed instructors for about twenty years. This often involved traveling to cities outside Minneapolis, including St. Cloud, Pipestone, and Duluth.

Pipestone

Pipestone, Minnesota is a small city in the southwestern part of Minnesota. The first time I went to the school, I drove out there by myself (over 205 miles, one-way.) I stopped at a gas station and asked where the Vo-Tech School was and the man said, "Just go down this street to where the old Murphy house burned down, turn right, go to the big oak tree and turn left, and it's in the old bowling alley." Now, if I had known where the Murphy House or the old bowling alley were located, I wouldn't have needed to ask directions!

The "Icy" Flight

After the first driving trip, I was usually flown to Pipestone. One time, the weather was really bad; ice was forming on the wings of the small plane. We could not see the ground.

Since Pipestone does not have a controlled airport, we had to go to Sioux Falls, South Dakota to be guided in by the control tower. We then could fly under the clouds and double back to Pipestone. When we landed, the pilot said, "You probably didn't notice, but we were icing up a little." Believe me, I noticed!

Supervising Student Teachers

Even though I was a nurse, I also supervised student teachers from St. Cloud State University. This mostly involved observing people teaching at Anoka TEC.

One particularly memorable observation involved a wood shop teacher, demonstrating how to use a lathe. He said, "This is turning really fast and it's really sharp, so you have to be careful not to push the wood against the blade too hard."

Suddenly, he dug too deep and a big piece of wood flew off, jetted to the back of the room, and crashed into the wall. And, all he said was, "See?" (We were fortunate it didn't hit anyone. He and I did have a little discussion after the students left the room.)

I could not have had any of these experiences had I not been a nurse educator.

There are many stories in the Naked City. I couldn't make up any of them.

CHAPTER 10

INTERIM POSITIONS, INCLUDING MINNESOTA LIONS' EYE BANK

This chapter is presented to further illustrate the myriad of employment opportunities, in addition to working in a hospital and teaching, which are open to nurses. I have held all these positions at some time during my nursing life. There are many more possibilities.

All these jobs increased my understanding of health care, human behavior, and probably most importantly, public relations. I have learned to work with people from all walks of life. My nursing background was helpful and/or necessary in all these positions.

Burke Marketing Research

Being Hired
After my second year in college (1957), I decided to stay in "the Cities" and work there. An ad in the paper for a marketing research job required a "college degree."

I went to the interview and they asked if I had a degree. I said "yes;" they asked what college and I said "the U." They didn't ask what type of degree, so I didn't tell them it was a two-year Associate Degree. They didn't ask to see a transcript. (Nobody had ever heard of a two-year college degree at that time.) The suggestion of my friend Barb to get the Associate Degree really paid off.

I told Burke I had some health care background and they were pleased with that, since we often tested health care products. So, they hired me.

Burke only found out my age when everyone was in a bar one day and I ordered a Coke. My friend and coworker Star-

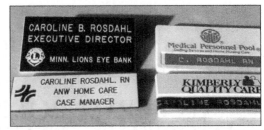

Name badges from interim nursing positions
(CB Rosdahl)

ia Walsh said, "You're not old enough to drink, are you?" I said I wasn't and she asked how I managed to get the job. After I explained, she acknowledged that I was already doing the work, so it was not a problem. (I don't think they ever told the owner of the company, however.)

This job was my introduction to the business world, which served me well later, particularly in Vocational Education.

Selection of Testing Sites

During the 1950s, many women were not working outside the home. They were generally home during the day and were usually happy to have someone to talk to. One part of the marketing research job involved going to homes and asking housewives about various products.

Sometimes, we had them try out two products and then on a return visit, tell us which they liked best and why. They were usually very cooperative. (I doubt if this method is used today, because most women are not home during the day. There might also be some danger to the researcher today.)

Most surveys were held in more than one city in the country. We mostly worked the Minneapolis/St. Paul area. The city being surveyed was divided into five zones, based on financial status. The top and most affluent economic zone (the "A" zone) was eliminated, because many of these people had cooks and/or maids. And, the bottom zone (the

"E" zone) was eliminated, because often these people were not home, because the area might be dangerous to us, or because the people were not able or willing to cooperate.

We then chose areas to survey at random, using equal numbers of B, C, and D homes. The way the areas were chosen was very primitive. First, a map of the city was laid flat. It was decided ahead of time how many areas would be surveyed. Then a specified number of nickels representing the zones were placed around, evenly spaced. The nickels were moved around to avoid lakes, rivers, parks, and other inappropriate areas.

Then, circles were drawn around the nickels and these were the target areas. We went only to single-family homes or duplexes, not apartments. Great effort was put into trying to obtain a representative sample of consumers who might be expected to use the products being tested.

Testing Products

We tested new food products like cooking oil and cereals. But, we also tested shampoo, toothpaste, pain relievers, face creams, and other health care products. Sometimes, a product was in two different sized bottles and we asked which contained the most. (They usually contained the same amount, but the bottles' shapes made one appear larger.)

One job involved new packaging for Lava Soap. The proposed wrapper had a picture of a volcano on the front, which took up almost the entire wrapper. *Not one person I interviewed made the connection between vol-*

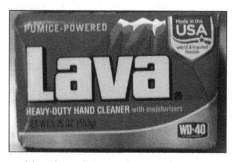

Most interviewees did not make the connection between the volcano and the name "LAVA" (CB Rosdahl)

cano and lava! Other people must have seen it though, because that wrapper was adopted and is still used today.

We also tested food items, such as cake mixes (which at that time were very new.) We worked for both Pillsbury *and* General Mills, major competitors, both located in the Twin Cities. We were sworn to secrecy, because of the competition for new products. We were also allowed to tour their facilities and see their ongoing research. (And, we met the lady who had been the model for "Betty Crocker.")

When we were testing a cake mix, for example, we would give the person two unlabeled cake mixes, without identifiers as to the manufacturer. The instructions for baking were on the box. We would ask the person to bake both cakes. Then, we would come back in a couple days and have the person answer questions about the time and ease of preparation and baking, and the taste of the product. We also asked about the clarity of the baking instructions. All this information was documented by hand; we did not have computers.

Burke Marketing Research gave me an Avis Rental Car to use. It was a new '57 Chevy hardtop convertible, white on red. I wish I still had it! I also got a chance to meet the owner of the company, which had its headquarters in Cincinnati, Ohio.

The Crash Landing and Visiting Chicago

That summer, I was sent to Chicago for a few weeks to do research on a particular shampoo. It was my *very first plane ride* and we *made a crash landing* at Midway Airport. Midway is surrounded by homes, unlike the newer O'Hare, which is further out of town.

The "crash" situation was caused by a faulty signal on the landing gear. The indicator did not show that the gear was locked down. So, we flew around and around the control tower. We could see people observing the plane through binoculars as we flew by.

They could see that the landing gear was down, but they couldn't decide if it was locked or not, so we made the crash landing. They foamed the runway, lined it with fire trucks and ambulances, and in we went!

We had to assume the *crash position as we came in.* We slid down the emergency slide to get out of the plane. (The gear *was locked down,* so we did not get hurt, but it was exciting.) I used some of my nursing skills that day to talk to other passengers. But, I had to think twice about getting back on a plane to go home.

We stayed at the Palmer House in downtown Chicago, which was very fancy at that time. Marilyn Monroe was also staying there. I rode in the elevator with her and she was not made up. (She looked just like the rest of us.) The hotel had stage shows in the dining room at night featuring various famous stars. We ate all our meals out and had time to visit the zoo, museums, and the beach.

We could have our laundry and hair done once a week and we could go home for the weekend every two weeks. We were on complete expense accounts, plus salary. Quite a deal for a poor twenty-year-old college student! And I was able to save some money.

The Interviews

The interviews in Chicago were done by phone, randomly calling people. The question was "What type of shampoo do you use and why?" Many people said they used Vaseline, lard, Shea butter, and other types of grease. And, most of the people said they were white.

Continuing in the Nursing Program

When we got home, the company wanted to send me to Texas. I had to admit that I was going back to school, so I could not travel any more. They offered to make me a manager, but I knew if I didn't go back to school then, I probably would never do so. This, of course, was *one of the best decisions of my life*. The company was very nice and allowed me to work part-time until I received my nursing cap the following March. (Chapter 2) Then I entered the clinical phase of the Nursing Program and did not have time to work there any longer.

The experience at Burke has been invaluable in my nursing career. Nurses can do anything!

Case Manager—Home Care

After leaving Anoka TEC, I tried out several nursing positions. I worked for a short time as a Case Manager for a home care agency. The work was interesting and I met many nice people. It was much like my Public Health experience. I enjoyed the clients, but the paper work was overwhelming. The more Medicare got involved, the worse it got. I decided that a record-keeping job was not for me and left after a few months.

Medical Personnel Pool and Kimberly

I also worked for two interim staffing services. This was very interesting, because I got a chance to work in many different healthcare facilities and every day was different. Usually, the staff at the facility was glad to see me, because I would help them out. Sometimes, they gave me the most difficult patients and that could be challenging. The work was much like my duties at General Hospital as the float nurse.

The Sad Charge Nurse

One day, I went to Orthopedics at St. Mary's Hospital in Minneapolis. The evening shift staff people were all in the report room and the day nurse came in, sat down, and began to cry. She had had a terrible day. That was scary, but we made it through the evening.

The Mental Health Unit

I was sent to a Psychiatric hospital, which had patients of all ages. One day, I cared for a little girl about eighteen months old. She was very psychotic. I asked how such a small child could be mentally ill and I was told that her father had been sexually abusing her. I could not imagine such a thing, particularly when the victim was a baby.

The "Rehabilitation" Center

I had told the agency that I would not go to a nursing home. One holiday (I think it was Thanksgiving), I was sent to a "Rehabilitation Center" in Minneapolis. I said this sounded like a nursing home and they said, "Oh, no, it's not." The agency lady said, "All I had to do was pass meds." When I got there, *I was the only nurse* and it was most definitely a nursing home. It was what we would call a "memory care" unit today.

There were several nursing assistants, many of whom did not speak English. There were about thirty or forty residents there, mostly elderly women, all with white hair and walkers or wheelchairs. Most of the residents were not wearing nametags and many of them did not know their own names. The nursing assistants did not seem to know the residents either and it was difficult to communicate with them.

I called the agency and said this was a nursing home and I was very upset. The lady at the agency said, "Well, if you don't like it, you can go home." Of course, *I could not go home*, because I was the only nurse! I made it through the day, but in good conscience I could not work for that agency any more.

Telephone Triage

I also did evening telephone triage for a national insurance company. People called from all over the country for assistance. I had to make a decision as to whether they should call an ambulance, go to an Emergency Room, or see their doctor the next day or later. Sometimes, I even had the responsibility of deciding if their insurance would pay for a particular treatment or not. This was often very difficult. (Some people even asked questions about their sick pets.)

I had lists of doctors in various cities and could refer people to them. We did not have computers, so *all the information was on a Rolodex file*. Sometimes, people had such a strong accent, it was difficult to understand them. Some of the questions they asked were bizarre.

The biggest problem with this job was the locality. I was all alone in a huge building at night. I don't think anyone else was in the building, except one custodian. I also missed being able to move around, because I had to be at the phone all the time. And, I missed being with people. I worked there a few months and it was good experience, but I did not want to do it long term.

Legal Consulting

I did a few legal cases for a local law firm. My job was to review accident cases and write up a report. In some cases, I had to do a deposition or testify in court. This was interesting, but a huge amount of work and research, which I found very tedious and I missed being with patients.

The Job Offer

As an aside, a few years ago I went to my doctor. He asked, "Are you ever going to retire?" I replied that "eventually" I would. He said, "When you retire, I would like you to come and do triage for me." I went home and told my family that I had gone to the doctor and also gotten a job offer. I really didn't want to do triage again, because I would rather work directly with people.

My Favorite Nursing Home Story

A few years after I moved to Mound, Minnesota in about 1988, I decided to try working in the local nursing home. There, I met a *106 year-old man* who was very sharp physically and mentally. He seemed to have no disabilities, except hearing loss. He said he "was just trying out the place to see if he liked it." He told about living in Mound when the roads were dirt and people drove horses and buggies.

The man was in such good shape, I was curious. I asked why he had decided to move onto a nursing home now and he said, "*I was living with my daughter and she got too old to take care of me!*" (I didn't ask, but she was probably in her eighties.) I didn't like nursing home work, partly because of the excessive paper work, and I only stayed there a short time.

Minnesota Lions' Eye Bank

I had the opportunity for a full-time job as Executive Director of the Minnesota Lions' Eye Bank. This was located in the Department of Ophthalmology at the University of Minnesota. This gave me a chance to explore a very interesting area of health care that was entirely new to me. I worked there for about two years. We were part of the National

Network of Eye Banks. We mostly sent corneas for transplant to Minnesota and the Dakotas, but sometimes, we sent them nationwide.

The eye bank obtained and processed corneas and other eye tissues for both corneal transplants and research. (If a person was under a certain age, the corneas could usually be used for transplant. If the person was older, they were used for research.)

We had certified staff people on call twenty-four hours a day; they did *enucleations* (removal of eyes after death). Some funeral directors were certified enucleators as well. In addition, the Red Cross and Life Source had people who could do enucleations, in combination with removal of other tissues or organs. Time is a factor; the eyes must be removed and taken to the laboratory within certain time limits.

Life Source and American Red Cross
We worked closely with Life Source, the agency responsible for obtaining body organs for transplantation. And we also worked closely with the American Red Cross, the Multi-Regional Tissue Bank. The Red Cross obtained bone, skin, heart valves, connective tissue, and other tissues for transplantation. (Some things have changed since I worked there.)

Community Relations
We did many presentations to hospitals and community organizations, to explain and promote organ and tissue donation. At that time, after a person died, their next-of-kin had to give permission for donation of organs and tissues, even though the person had designated him/herself as a donor. (This is no longer true in all cases.)

We often met with hospital personnel and families to discuss donation. We gave speeches at meetings and conferences. It was important for families and healthcare staff to realize that eye donation and donation of organs and tissues does not cause disfigurement.

The Eye Bank Advisory Committee was made up of Lions Club members. They were very helpful and supportive and assisted in publicizing the value of donation. For example, the Lions had a booth at the

Minnesota State Fair and we helped staff the booth. We also co-sponsored memorial tree-plantings and other events with Life Source and the Red Cross, honoring donors and recipients.

National Conferences

We went to a couple national Eye Bank conferences, one in Marco Island, Florida, and one in Portland, Oregon. At these conferences, we had very interesting speakers and got a chance to meet professionals from all over the country. They also had displays of many different pieces of medical equipment and medications.

Sometimes, recipients would give a speech about their experiences and were able to describe how their life had changed since receiving the donated tissue or organ. In some cases, donor families and recipients were able to meet. This was a very emotional experience.

These national conferences were a very bright spot in my time of employment at the Eye Bank. I met many nice people and learned a lot more about donation and transplantation.

The Medical Director

The Medical Director, in his early professional life had developed several innovative methods and products to be used in corneal transplantation. He had been at the University for many years. However, now it was difficult for him to listen to anyone else's point of view.

The Broken Leg

I broke my leg while I worked there and the Director's greatest concern was "how much work would I miss?" (I only missed two days to have surgery.) When I returned, I was non-weight-bearing. At that time, there were no facilities for "handicapped" people, so it was quite challenging.

I am sure I was driving illegally, but I would put my casted right leg up on the car's center console and drive with my left foot. I used a wheelchair to transport myself and my "stuff" up to the office. Then, I "crutched" around the Eye Bank department. I was given a parking space in the lower level of the building, but there was no power door to help me get into the elevator lobby. And, there was one step to navigate, no ramp. It was interesting to figure out how to manage, but I learned a lot about how difficult it is to have a disability. (The first wheelchair I rented had a broken wheel; it would only go in circles. It took me a while to figure out it was not my driving, but the wheelchair that was defective.)

I have discovered that the United States has made great advancements to accommodate people with disabilities. (This is often not true in other countries.)

Reasons for Leaving

There were two "final straws" that led me to look for other employment. The first occurred while my husband and I were camping in the mountains on the West Coast. I had been told to call the Eye Bank every few days, since there were no cell phones then.

As soon as I got out of the mountains, I called. I was on top of a mountain at a rest stop, calling from an outside pay phone, next to a running semi truck. So, I could barely hear. I was told that I "had to come back right away." I said I couldn't and the Director yelled at me and said I had to. I figured he would calm down by the time I got back, but he didn't. There had been an error related to the removal of eyes. This was terrible, but obviously there was nothing I could do about it then, even if I came right back. (Even if I had been there when the incident occurred, I would not have been able to do anything about it. The Director just wanted someone to blame.)

I asked if this meant I couldn't ever go camping and I was told that *I had to tell the Eye Bank where I was at all times and had to have phone service at all times, day and night.* I would not be allowed to go camping, canoeing, or backpacking in a remote area as long as I was employed by the Eye Bank. *Even if I was on a regularly scheduled vacation!*

The final, final straw was when I was ordered to fire one of the employees. I said I would do an evaluation, which I did. I also said I would follow appropriate and legal steps for evaluation and termination, if that was warranted. The employee had been with the Eye Bank for a number of years, much longer than I had been there.

I did the employee evaluation and there were some areas for improvement, but termination was certainly not appropriate. I wrote up a "Plan of Assistance," discussed it with the employee and got a signature. I then turned the evaluation in to the Director.

The next day, *the Director's secretary* called me and said, "I won't accept this evaluation." I told her it was not up to her to accept or reject and that it was a fair evaluation, discussed and signed by the employee. The Director called me in and demanded that I fire the employee. I replied, "That is not appropriate or legal. You will have my resignation as soon as I can type it."

When I presented my letter of resignation to the Director, he said, "You will never find another job at your age!" (Fifty-three.) What he didn't know was that I already had another job offer (Hennepin County Medical Center) and I later *worked there for almost twenty-six years.* I didn't tell anyone in the Eye Bank where I was going, because I figured the Eye Bank would try to sabotage me.

My Friend was Smarter than I Was

I found out later that a good friend of mine had also applied for the Eye Bank job. She was very grateful she didn't get it when she heard the stories. I am not sorry I worked there, because I really learned a lot. And I made a couple of good friends. But I also was not sorry to leave.

A Writing Opportunity

While I was at the Eye Bank, I was asked to write a section of an Ophthalmology Surgery Textbook. (See Bibliography) This chapter related to cooperative relationships between donation agencies. It was a great honor to have been asked to write a portion of this prestigious book. I was surprised the Director didn't force me to make him a co-author. All of these positions added to my life experience. I had an opportunity to meet many people from all walks of life. I am grateful that I had this experience.

And, again this proves that nurses have many choices and can do many different things. And, again I was exposed to more and different adventures in the "Naked City."

CHAPTER 11

WRITING EXPERIENCES

Many nurses would like to be writers. We have so many stories to share. There are several venues for nurse authors. Nurses write journal articles, newspaper stories, self-study continuing education modules, workshops, TV stories, and nursing textbooks. This can be full time or part time. If you always have wanted to write, go for it!

As I said in the Acknowledgment, my father, Frank Bunker, was a poet. I wrote my first poem at age five. I always thought I would enjoy being a writer, particularly since I was from the same town (Sauk Centre, Minnesota) as the famous author, Sinclair Lewis.

But, I actually became a writer through a series of fortunate accidents. This current book is my first authorship of anything other than a nursing article or a textbook.

This chapter relates many of the stories and adventures I had while writing and traveling for my books. I would never have had these opportunities if I had not first been a nurse.

Bennett Books, Peoria, Illinois

Often, writing opportunities come about unexpectedly, as in my case. One day while I was working at Anoka TEC, a book salesman named Mike Kenney approached me. (Chapter 7)

He asked, "You're a nurse. Right? Are you also child development expert?"

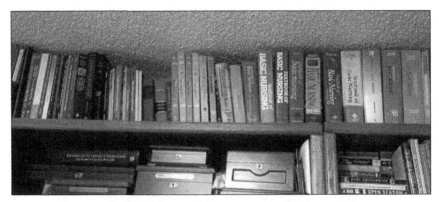

Books by Caroline Bunker Rosdahl (CB Rosdahl)

I thought he was joking, so I said, "Of course I am."

He was looking for someone to write a new child development chapter for the revision of an existing high school Home Economics book, *Homemaking for Teenagers*. (See Bibliography) I had never written material for a book before. I had written a few journal articles. Mike asked if I would be interested.

I figured, from my "vast" experience as a nurse and the mother of a small child, I could do research as well as anyone. So, I agreed to write the chapter.

I had never had classes related to writing, either in high school or college. Therefore, writing the chapter turned out to be a very valuable and educational experience, since Mike was an excellent editor. He helped me a great deal along the way. He encouraged my research and taught me how to format and organize material.

Mike also advised me how to obtain art and the related permissions. In addition to photos obtained from commercial sources, I was able to use photos of my son, Keith, and photos of my friends' children. It is fun to look at the chapter now and see these early photos of young children who are now in their fifties. In addition, a friend asked her nephew Paul Barke to draw a couple of custom illustrations for the book.

The Jamaica Trip

I was paid a total of $600 for doing the Child Development chapter.

This amounted to probably about ten cents an hour. But in those days (1971), it was enough to *fully pay for a seven-day cruise* to Jamaica for my husband and myself.

The Bad News

Mike also became a friend. His wife had cancer and they had a couple of very young children. Because I was a nurse, I became Mike's "nursing consultant." He would call me after taking his wife to the doctor. He would tell me what the doctor had said and ask what that meant. *It was all bad news*, but I tried to be as positive as possible.

Mike's wife did die and Mike later married a woman who had been a Catholic nun. She said she "felt she had a higher calling, to raise Mike's little children." As far as I know, they are still married. I have not talked to Mike for many years.

J.B. Lippincott, Philadelphia PA

This company has been sold several times. Later names include: Lippincott Williams & Wilkins (LWW); LWW/WoltersKluwer, and now simply, WoltersKluwer. (The main headquarters of WoltersKluwer is in the Netherlands.) For many years, it was family-owned.

Measurable Behavioral Objectives

Chapter 7 describes the development of behavioral objectives in the PN Program at Anoka. These were the first in the U.S. and, I believe, first in the world. They are now used in nursing programs at all levels. Behavioral objectives allow students to know exactly what is expected of them and the instructors to accurately measure student performance.

The Beginning of *Textbook of Basic Nursing*

Lippincott found out about the objectives and contacted me. They wanted me to write a book for them. I was super busy and did not have time, but Lippincott hounded me for about a year. They had seen my writing in the Home Economics book and had also seen the course outlines I had written for Anoka.

Lippincott's book *Simplified Nursing*, was originally intended to teach Practical Nurses. That book was first copyrighted in 1925 and had gone through several editions. It had become much too basic for Practical Nurses. The company wanted to break this book into two books, one for Nursing Assistants

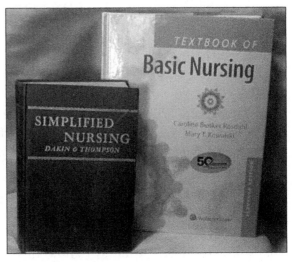

Simplified Nursing, compared to *Textbook of Basic Nursing* (CB Rosdahl)

and one for Practical Nurses. As a matter of fact, I had used it when I taught nursing assistant students at Hopkins High School. (Chapter 4)

Had I not been a nurse, I would never have seen this book before.

A person was hired by Lippincott to split this book, but she did not complete her assignment, so in haste, the book was split by Lippincott editors. This was the first edition of *Textbook of Basic Nursing* in 1966. Finally after being begged by Lippincott, I agreed to take on the project. Thus, I have written ten more editions of this textbook (and the 12th Edition is being planned.) *Simplified Nursing* was 800+ pages; the eleventh edition of *Textbook of Basic Nursing* is over 2,000 pages.

It would be impossible to recognize that the recent editions were based on

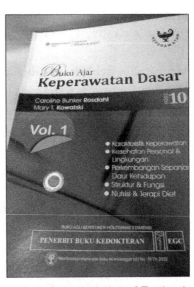

Indonesian translation of *Textbook of Basic Nursing*, Volume One (CB Rosdahl)

the original book. They do not resemble it in any way. Nursing has become much more complex and detailed, and practical nurses have so many added responsibilities. Many photos (now in color) have been added, as well as teaching hints, study questions, and of course, more detailed behavioral objectives. In addition, there are workbooks, test banks, teachers' guides, and other materials to accompany the books. There is also an electronic version of the book, as well as other on-line materials to assist students. (*And, now there is an Indonesian translation, published in five volumes.*)

The 50th Anniversary Edition of the Book

The editions of *Textbook of Basic Nursing* are listed in Appendix C. The 2017 Edition is being marketed as the "50th Anniversary Edition."

Obtaining Illustrations

It was wonderful that 3M (Minnesota Mining and Manufacturing), located in the Twin Cities, helped me with illustrations for earlier editions. Had I not been a nurse, they would never have allowed me to do that. I was able to go through all their Health Product Division photo files and choose the ones I wanted to use. They printed them for me, without charge. In addition, most of the time, using these files allowed me to obtain illustrations without having to obtain permissions.

Later, I was also able to use Lippincott file photos. As time progressed, we made sure to have people from all races in the photos. We also show male nurses. And nurses are mostly wearing scrubs, rather than white uniforms. In some cases, nurses are shown in their traditional religious-based clothing and head covering. Nearly all the photos in the book are in full color.

My First Computer

My first edition of the book was written out in longhand. I had a secretary type it. Then, I went through it and made changes and additions and she typed it again. Later, we got an electronic typewriter, which made things a little easier.

I had never had a computer course in nursing classes, but I had to learn. My husband and I built a computer, using a "Heath Kit." This computer was very large and cumbersome. As time went on, we obtained a regular tower computer and eventually, a laptop. Much of the material for the book is now submitted in digital format, eliminating the need to print out the chapters.

In about 2005, we got computers at Hennepin County Medical Center. It turned out that I was almost the only person on the staff who had ever used one before. (Chapter 12)

Contributors and Consultants

I hired many consultants over the years to assist in writing the book. In areas that were not my specialties, I hired contributors to write that chapter or section of the book. I then rewrote much of the material, to keep the style consistent. I have met many wonderful and skilled nurses and other healthcare specialists from all over the country and I am grateful to all of them for their assistance. Some of them have gone on to write materials on their own for publication.

Trips to Philadelphia versus Conference Calls

During the early years of writing the textbook, I had to travel to Lippincott in Philadelphia fairly often. Now, this is done via conference calls. On one of my visits to the home office, I had the opportunity to meet Barton Lippincott, the last member of the family to be associated with the company. He was a tall man and he was very pleasant. It was a great honor to meet him.

An Excellent Decision

Taking on this project was, in retrospect, a very good decision. I have learned so much and have been forced to keep up with current trends in nursing. I have met many notable and brilliant people. I have learned about newly discovered illnesses, new equipment and medications, and new procedures. It has certainly has helped me to keep up to date. The book has been a great deal of work, (impossible to describe—thousands of hours), but it has been very rewarding. Every edition, I say I will not do it again. But, one never knows . . ..

McGraw-Hill, New York City

The National Advisory Committee

I had many adventures while working for McGraw-Hill, based totally on the fact that I was a nurse and an author. First, I was named to their National Advisory Committee on High School Health Careers. We held the first meeting at the McGraw-Hill headquarters in Rockefeller Center in New York City. Members of the committee included: Nancy from the Carolinas; Diane Watson from California; Karl Wittman, Health Occupations Supervisor for New York State; Helen Powers, Health Careers Consultant from the U.S. Department of Education; Joe Bonnice, from McGraw-Hill; and myself, as well as representatives from other states, including Texas, Oregon, and Illinois. Being on this committee allowed me to meet these nationally influential people.

The task of this Advisory Committee was to plan and oversee the development of a series of health careers books for high school students. These books were designed to teach students various entry-level health occupations.

I was later hired as the Consultant to the total McGraw-Hill "Nursing and Allied Health Series" of books. My job was to plan the books to be included, locate authors, supervise the development of the books, and serve as Editor. McGraw-Hill published seven titles, plus ancillaries, which I supervised. These books are listed In Appendix C.

Adventures with McGraw-Hill

We had many adventures while working for McGraw-Hill. The office was high up in the Rockefeller Center in Midtown Manhattan. Just being there was an adventure for me, since I had not been in New York City before.

The Hotel Fire

While we were in New York for our *first Advisory Committee meeting*, there was a fire in our hotel. We had been out to dinner, so we were not involved in the actual fire. However, we were not allowed to re-enter the hotel when we got back. So, the company had to find an alternate hotel for us. Here we were, with only the clothes on our backs. We went over to Grand Central Station and got toothbrushes, toothpaste, and deodorant out of vending machines. Our rooms were all in a row, so we shared some things, such as toothpaste.

As we were watching the fire, Diane said, "My best boots are in there." Nancy said in her very strong Southern accent, "My husband is coming for the weekend and my birth control pills are in there." (I told her to call me when she got home and tell me if everything was okay.)

The next day we were all wearing the same clothes we had been wearing the previous day. After a couple of days, the Fire Department let us go back into our old hotel to get our stuff. We had to be accompanied by a police officer. When I got to my room, the door had been chopped through with an ax. (The firemen had to make sure nobody was in there.) It was a very creepy feeling. We couldn't wear our clothes, since they still smelled very strongly of smoke. So, the company gave us money to buy new underwear and clothes. They also paid to have our clothes dry-cleaned when we got home. It was quite an adventure.

"I Have Nothing to Tell You"

The funniest thing happened about a month later. My secretary came into my office and said, "You got the weirdest phone call. A lady with a strong Southern accent called and said, '*I am calling you to tell you I have nothing to tell you.*'" My secretary asked me, "Does this mean anything to you?" I told her it did. (It meant that Nancy was not pregnant.)

Marketing Conferences

As the nurse editor of the Nursing and Health Careers Series, I was asked to speak at company marketing conferences. All the marketing representatives were men with no health background. I had to be there as the nursing representative to explain some of the materials and how they could be used with students.

Many of the people from New York weren't sure if anyone living west of Philadelphia (except California) could function in "polite society," so I had to prove myself. The person who organized my speaking tours was Marvin. Marv was very nervous, insecure, and concerned about appearances. He really was not quite sure if I, the naïve girl from the Midwest, would be able to behave appropriately at these meetings. So, he quizzed me and watched over me, to make sure I didn't embarrass him.

The Bicentennial Tour

My son, Keith, was able to go with me on a tour during the bicentennial year of 1976, when he was ten years old. Cities on this tour included Philadelphia, Boston, and Syracuse. On the way out, we flew over Saranac Lake, about a hundred miles from Stowe, Vermont. As we were flying over the lake, we suddenly dropped about 500 feet. I was terrified. Keith thought it was fun and yelled, "Whoopie!" (Oh, the innocence of a child!)

We stopped to go skiing at Stowe, Vermont. (Snow conditions: *"Bare to glare, with a bulletproof base."*) The runs were very icy and you could see rocks through the ice. There was a sheer drop-off on the right. Keith took off and I hardly saw him the rest of the day. He had no fear. At Stowe, Keith had fondue for the first time in his life. He thought that was great fun.

In Philadelphia, I hired a nanny to spend the day taking Keith to all the historic sites. She said, "He was having so much fun at the Science Museum that I practically had to drag him out of there." We ate dinner at the Rusty Scupper, where the menu was printed on a small canoe paddle. Keith, of course, had to have one.

The Bunker Hill Monument and the Canoe Paddle

We then went to Boston and the conference there, and then we went on to Syracuse. McGraw-Hill had made plane reservations for us from

Boston to Syracuse on Pilgrim Airlines, which I had never heard of. The plane was small, with only four passengers, including us. The rest of the seats had been removed to make room for bags of mail and boxes of freight. The pilot had a thermos of coffee and some cups and he turned around and asked if we wanted any.

Keith told the pilot his middle name was Bunker, so the pilot let Keith sit in the co-pilot's seat and we flew around the Bunker Hill Monument several times. (The FAA would never let him do that today.)

One of the McGraw-Hill salesmen was to meet us in Syracuse. When I told him I was coming in on Pilgrim Airlines, he had never heard of it either. The salesman asked how he would recognize me at the Syracuse airport and I told him I was with a ten-year-old boy carrying a canoe paddle. He had no difficulty recognizing us!

King of Prussia, Pennsylvania

On another trip, I was told that the conference was to be in place called "King of Prussia." I asked where in the world that was. I had never heard of it. *I didn't even know what state it was in.* They said, "Just fly to Philadelphia and take a shuttle."

At this conference, I had a free afternoon and wanted to go sightseeing. One of the men said I could use his company car and gave me his car keys. The only problem was, all the company cars were identical! There were no fobs with beepers at that time, so I just walked around the parking lot, trying the keys in all the cars. It wasn't long before the hotel security guard approached me and asked what was going on. I told him, "I'm looking for the car that fits this key." After I explained, he helped me, and eventually I found the car.

I particularly enjoyed visiting some of George Washington's haunts, especially Valley Forge National Historical Park. (Today, I would probably be arrested at gunpoint by the hotel guard.)

New Orleans, Louisiana

Another trip took me to New Orleans. While there, I got the twenty-four-hour stomach flu. When I was feeling better, I went into a restaurant and ordered *dark toast* and tea. The server brought me white toast. I said I really needed dark toast, so she took it back into the kitchen and they toasted it several more times, until it was burned black.

No Ham and Eggs
Another time, I ordered ham and eggs for breakfast.

The waitress said, "I can't serve that to you." I asked if they were out of ham and she said, "No."

I asked if they were out of eggs and she said, "No."

I then asked what the problem was and she said, "We're out of grits." She explained that they served grits with everything and it was considered a necessary garnish. When I finally convinced her I didn't need grits, I got my ham and eggs. (I don't even like grits.)

"Girls" in the Middle of the Night
The funniest thing that happened in New Orleans occurred about four A.M. Several of us (the guys and I) were in the beignet place in the French Quarter. (A beignet is a sugary doughnut-like thing.) Four beautiful girls, dressed fit to kill, came in. The guys got very interested and I said, "Be careful. They may not be girls."

Being a nurse and a woman, I could tell they were female impersonators in drag, just leaving their performance at a local nightclub. They could have fooled people, particularly from the distance of a stage. The "boys" I was with would have been very surprised if they had taken one of these "girls" home!

Other Marketing Conferences
I also did marketing conferences in cities like Huntington, West Virginia (where we also toured the glass factory); Los Angeles, California; and Lafayette, Louisiana.

While driving from Memphis to Lafayette at night, there were miles and miles with no lights or any sign of civilization. On the way back,

I discovered that it was a huge lowland area and indeed nobody lived there. (Good thing I didn't have car trouble.)

The Florida Conference

One of the marketing conferences was at a fancy golf resort in Central Florida. Marv called me a couple weeks before the conference to make sure I had a plane reservation. I told him I had a non-stop flight into Orlando. He said, "Oh, you are flying to Chicago and then catching a non-stop flight?"

I said, "No, we have a little *hometown airline* called Norwest Orient and I have a non-stop from Minneapolis." He couldn't believe it.

The Bowling Shirt

A few days later, Marv called and told me the resort we were going to was really fancy and he wanted to make sure I would be dressed appropriately. I said, "Oh, I have a new bowling shirt and it has my name on it and everything. So, I won't need a name tag." Guess who met me at the airport in Florida? (Marv spent a lot of time worrying that I would embarrass him, because I was from the "boonies." I probably drove him nuts.)

Because of Marv's warning, I had brought many changes of clothes, not knowing how other people would be dressed. I hung them in the closet of my room and went down to the swimming pool. I found that it was *very hot* and all the salesmen were wearing golf shirts and shorts. Only Marv was wearing a suit, white shirt, and tie. So, I managed to fit in!

The New Roommate

I was swimming around in the pool and suddenly I saw two feet standing at the edge of the pool. A man I didn't know was there and he said, "Hi. I'm your new roommate." This happened because the hotel had been given only last names and they just paired up the McGraw-Hill guests, not knowing I was a woman. This salesman said he didn't know what to do when he got into the room and saw women's clothes, because he was afraid one of the guys had brought his wife or girl friend. Of course, I was given my own room, but it was funny.

The Golf Tournament

One day, the guys were planning to have a golf tournament and they invited me to join them. When I went to the Pro Shop to rent clubs, I was told the price of the golf. I thought it was *terribly expensive* (probably equivalent to about $500-600 today). I asked about this and the Pro said the price *included a golf cart and caddy.*

I was young and I said, "I don't need a golf cart." And, he said, "Yes you do."

I then said, "I don't need a caddy, especially if I have a cart." And, he said, "Yes, you do."

I asked why and he went on to tell me that the cart would keep me up off the ground, so I wouldn't be attacked by poisonous snakes. And the caddy knew where the alligators were if I hit a ball into the swamp. And he would know which snakes were poisonous.

I decided I didn't want to play golf that badly!

The California Trip

Marv and I went to California to meet with Diane Watson, one of our authors. Diane is about six-foot-two (without heels) and she is a very dark-skinned black woman. She and I made an interesting pair, since I am just over five feet tall and white. One night Diane took us to a nightclub where a friend of hers, Barbara McNair (who was quite famous at the time), was singing. Marv was totally star-struck. We went backstage to meet the singer and Marv could hardly speak.

Diane's Accomplishments

Diane eventually earned a PhD and was a school psychologist in Los Angeles. Marv would have been very impressed with her PhD. What Marv probably didn't know what that Diane was the first African-American woman to become a California State Senator. And later in 1998,

President Clinton appointed Diane to be Ambassador to the Federated States of Micronesia. She later served in the U.S. House of Representatives from 2001 until she retired in 2011 to care for her 100-year-old mother. (Diane was on the House Foreign Affairs Committee and the House Oversight and Government Reform Committee.) Diane was a very impressive woman and a wonderful friend. (Marv would have been totally shocked had he known what else Diane had done with her life after working with us at McGraw-Hill.)

Other McGraw-Hill Stories

Rooftop Photo
On one trip, the company decided to take a publicity photo of me on the roof of Rockefeller Center with the city in the background. This roof is not designed for public access, so there is just a small parapet (barrier) about a foot high at the edge. The photographer kept telling me to "back up some more." I was really afraid I would fall off. And, it was so windy that day, the photos made me look like a wild woman, so they were never used.

The Cocktail Party
There was a *very fancy* cocktail party at the McGraw-Hill headquarters to introduce new products, including the High School Health Occupations Series. They had me come to New York specifically for this party. Marv took me to the party, *after checking to make sure I was appropriately dressed.*

A large crowd was at the party and Marv seemed overwhelmed. The President of the company, Don Fruehling, was there of course. Marv was very nervous, because he had only met Mr. Fruehling very briefly once before and that was in a big group. *Marv was trying to decide if he had the nerve to introduce me.*

Suddenly, a voice from across the room yelled, "*Rosdahl, what are you doing here?*" It was a teacher friend from Hopkins High School, Rosemary Shanus (Fruehling). She had recently married Mr. Fruehling. I did not know about this and she did not realize I had been on the National Advisory Committee or had managed the publication of the High School series. We had a fun reunion and she took me to meet her new husband, Don.

Insecure Marv was totally overwhelmed and flummoxed. He could not believe I knew the wife of his company's President. It's a small world and nurses are everywhere!

Sexual Harassment

We have all heard stories about sexual harassment and about traveling salesmen. Unfortunately, many of these stories were true at that time. I was hustled, but I never had any trouble I couldn't handle. However, I can't imagine being married to one of those guys.

One of the men found out that his wife had had enough when he went home one day. The wife had put all his belongings out on the curb in front of their house and she was selling everything. He said, "I didn't even have a suitcase to pack my clothes in. She sold them all!"

The Restaurant

Marv really believed that Minnesota was very uncivilized and backward. Many times, he made comments that struck me as funny. Once when I was in New York, he said, "I am going to take you to a special restaurant. I am sure you don't have anything like it in Minnesota." He took me to *TGI Friday's*, which has *several locations* in the Twin Cities and throughout Minnesota.

The Elevators

Another time, when Marv was visiting Minneapolis, I took him to a restaurant at the top of the IDS Building. When we entered the lobby, Marv said, "Oh, you have elevators here just like in New York." I knew he meant elevators that go from 1-29 and 30-49, but it sounded ridiculous the way he said it.

The Job Offer

Marv could not understand why I didn't want to move to New York. He could not believe that I was making much more money in Minnesota than I would have made in New York. (I had to show him my contract to prove it.) In addition, living expenses were far higher in New York.

The Boat Hitch

A group of the McGraw-Hill salesmen were in Minnesota for a conference. The company had them located at the Lafayette Club, which is fairly far out of town, thinking they could not leave and would have to stay there and work. The guys called me and begged me to pick them up. They said they would take me to dinner anywhere I wanted to go.

When I picked them up, they looked at my car and asked, "Is that a boat hitch?" I said it was a *trailer hitch*. They asked if I had a boat and I said I did.

They said, "In New York, if someone buys a car, they put a boat hitch on it, just so people will think they have a boat." (Most people in New York City do not even have a car, because the traffic is so terrible and parking is extremely expensive.)

Miscellaneous Writing

All my writing has been related to nursing and healthcare. I believe my varied work experiences and my education prepared me for these writing experiences. A complete listing of my publications appears in Appendix C.

"Oh, you're the book!"

I was at a conference years ago and a lady was introduced to me.

She said, "But you're so young!" (People don't say that any more.)

Another time a lady read my nametag and exclaimed, "*Oh my, you're the book!*"

There is no limit to the types of work a nurse can do. Follow your dream!

CHAPTER 12

PSYCHIATRY/MENTAL HEALTH AT HCMC

My First Introduction to Mental Illness

When I was very young, I took piano lessons from Miss W. at her home. When I was there, I often heard someone walking around upstairs. I asked my father about this and he explained the situation. (He had lived in the town for years, so he knew everyone.) Miss W's brother was mentally ill, which at that time was considered a disgrace. (He was in his forties.) The family was embarrassed and didn't want anyone to know about it. So, it was a big secret.

This man had been kept isolated his entire life. He was kept upstairs at all times and was never allowed to go outside. He had no friends, no stimulation, and no education. (The only alternative for him was the "Insane Asylum," where conditions were very undesirable.) Most of the people in town had never seen this man and, in fact, most people did not even know he existed. They certainly were not aware of his illness.

There was a very strong stigma about mental illness at that time. Public education today has caused some improvement, but mental illness is still considered by many to be a cause for shame or fear. If a person has a physical illness, that person is treated kindly. People ask how they are doing and offer to help. In too many situations, the person with a mental disorder is avoided and ignored and is not treated kindly. People may also be afraid of them.

Hearing about this young man when I was very young made a great impression on me. I vowed never to shun these people and to try to help them. I have met many people with psychological disorders during my entire career. I hope I have helped at least some of them. Working on a Mental Health Unit presents unique challenges for the nurse and I loved it.

My Interview at Hennepin County Medical Center (HCMC/ HHC)

In 1991, when I went in to interview for the position at HCMC, I was asked to wait in the lounge outside the offices. There were several people there. I am sure they were clients waiting to be seen. I also think I may have been observed from the offices, to see how I related to these people.

I was interviewed by John Gray the Supervisor, and his assistant, Lucy Fallon. I had worked with Lucy in Anoka. I am sure she recommended me for the job. I was hired immediately. It's a small world!

The Truth About Mental Illness

I need to repeat some of what I stated elsewhere in the book, with an emphasis on mental illness. Mental Illness is not funny. It is serious and may be life-threatening. It affects not only the patient/client, but also the entire family.

Some situations are humorous, but some are very sad. I do not in any way intend to insult or demean anyone with these stories. But, observing human nature can help us gain insight into the workings of the human mind.

And, sometimes a little humor can help defuse a very uncomfortable situation. Of course, a person does not need to be in a Mental Health Unit to say or do unusual, humorous, or interesting things.

In addition, it is important to remember that many clients in areas of the hospital *other than Psychiatry* have mental health issues. These concerns are not exclusive to clients in just the inpatient Mental Health Units.

It is also very important to remember that *most people with mental health concerns are not in the hospital.* Many of these people in the community function very well with the assistance of medications and counseling.

Treatments and Care of Persons with Mental Health Concerns

Psych Medications

Many clients with mental health concerns are on medications. Some of the medications have very undesirable side effects or are very expensive, so the person stops taking them.

This is one of the reasons that clients come into the hospital. They get back on their medications to get regulated, go home, then stop the medications, and return again to the hospital. This situation is known as *chronic and persistent mental illness* (CPMI.) Unfortunately, there is not enough support in the community to prevent some of these re-hospitalizations.

Other people come into the hospital once, get regulated, and we never see them again. These are the reassuring cases.

The Mental Health Units at Hennepin Healthcare

When I left the Eye Bank, I was interviewed for a position at HCMC in the Psych (Mental Health) Units. I told them I was already retired (from Education), but I promised to stay "at least a year or two." However, I ended up working there for nearly twenty-six years.

There are six Mental Health Units at HCMC (now called Hennepin Healthcare—HHC). Four are general Psychiatric units and two are Psych Intensive Care Units (ICUs.) In the ICUs, people with more severe illness or those who might be assaultive are usually located. The Psych units all are locked, with sally port entrances to help prevent elopement (escape.)

The sally ports are similar to those in a jail. There is an outside door with a vestibule, called a *sally port*. Then, there is an inner door, which cannot be opened until the outside door is closed. (This works in reverse when leaving the unit.) The people on Psych/Mental Health units are often referred to as "clients," to help them to feel more normal.

Physical Disorders

In many cases, clients in Mental Health Units have physical illnesses or injuries. So, in addition to mental health issues, psych nurses deal with medical treatments. These include IVs; administering PPDs, diabetic insulin and other injections; and clients having blood tests, x-rays, MRIs, or other tests. Some clients are on special diets. Some need dressing changes. Some have mobility issues and are in traction or using wheelchairs. Some people have surgery and are returned immediately to the Psych unit.

Psych nurses also deal with many people who are seriously overweight, because some of the medications cause people to gain weight. In some cases, prescribed medications also contribute to kidney disease, diabetes, and other physical disorders, as well as a movement disorder called *tardive dyskinesia*.

Dual Disorders

Many clients in Mental Health Units have another disorder, in addition to their mental health issues. These are called *dual disorders*. One of the most common of the dual disorders is mental illness combined with chemical dependency (MI-CD.) It is easy to understand why a person with serious mental health issues becomes chemically dependent.

Drugs are often taken to offset auditory or visual *hallucinations* (hearing voices or seeing things that are not there) or just to relieve some of the anxiety and confusion the client has. It is also very easy to become addicted to pain and anti-anxiety medications, as well as alcohol.

Other dual disorders often seen in Mental Health Units include eating disorders, sexual deviance, and other adjustment disorders.

These dual disorders may be treated together or as two or more separate illnesses.

Smoking

When I first started working at HCMC, clients were allowed to smoke in the common lounge. Later, they were given a special room, the "Smoker." The accrediting agency then notified the hospital that our accreditation would be revoked unless smoking was totally discontinued.

Our hospital continued to allow clients to smoke until the very last minute, but we were finally forced to discontinue the practice. This was difficult, because nearly all the clients smoked. It gave them a little comfort and relaxation and was a social time for them. Some people refused to come to our hospital when smoking was discontinued, but they soon learned that other hospitals would not allow them to smoke either.

When smoking was discontinued, people still occasionally managed to get a cigarette from a visitor or had some hidden in their rooms. Then, they had to find innovative ways to light their cigarettes. Some tried using the toaster, which was a good way to start a fire, but not a great way to light a cigarette.

Some tried to use electrical outlets, which was really dangerous. One man tried to use the microwave. This smelled up the entire unit, but did not light the cigarette. Now, people hardly ever try to sneak a smoke, because it has become so difficult.

One man lit his mattress on fire with hidden matches while he was restrained in bed. Staff people had to risk their lives to rescue him. (One rescuer was seriously burned in this incident.)

Safety

Attempts have been made to make Mental Health units as safe as possible. Many changes were made during the time I worked there. For example, all the windows on the units are plexiglass and only open at the very top, near the ceiling. Clients are not allowed to have shoelaces, belts, drawstrings, plastic bags, or other items that could be used to harm themselves. Some clients are required to wear hospital pajamas all the time, for their own safety. (Most clients wear street clothes, to help them feel as normal as possible and to prepare them to return to society.)

Suicide Risk

Many people with mental health issues become suicidal. Often, they make a suicide attempt and are not successful. Then, these people are usually admitted to the Mental Health unit. In some cases, extensive surgical repair or other treatments are needed. If a person comes into the Crisis Center saying they are feeling suicidal, even if they have not made an attempt, they are usually admitted to the inpatient unit (on a seventy-two hour hold) for observation and evaluation.

Gunshot Wounds

If a person tries to shoot himself or herself, the wounds are usually very severe. In addition to counseling, the person often requires many surgeries, to repair the damage.

Other Suicide Attempts

Many other methods are used to attempt suicide. These include hanging, cutting oneself, taking pills, using carbon monoxide, or drinking a caustic substance. Often they say, "The voices told me to do it." The clients' injuries are treated symptomatically. For example, carbon monoxide victims are often treated in the Hyperbaric Chamber. (Chapter 5)

Sometimes, clients lie and say they are not suicidal so they can get out of the hospital. This was the case of the social worker described in Chapter 5.

One Day, I walked past a gentleman's room and he was in bed, with his head covered up with bedding. Something just didn't look right, so I went in to check. He had tied a plastic bag around his head. I ripped it open, just in time. He had no serious after-effects. Fortunately, plastic bags were later banned from the units.

One day, a coworker passed the shower and just had a feeling that something was wrong. She entered the shower to find a client who had hanged himself. She called for help and held him up until others came. He was cut down and he lived. Had she not rescued him when she did, he would have completed the suicide. (The nurse was pregnant at the time, so lifting the client was very difficult.)

In some cases, a person will deliberately commit a crime in an attempt to have the police shoot him or her. You have probably heard this called "suicide by cop."

I have talked to a number of people who were happy they did not succeed with a suicide attempt. People often say they are very happy they are alive and will never do anything like that again. They go on to live a functioning and productive life. And we never see them again.

Assault Risk and Staff Safety

In rare cases, clients with mental health issues are violent. These people are the *extreme minority*. (*Most clients are more dangerous to themselves than they are to others*.) I always felt quite safe, because I am a "little old lady" and not a physical threat. The staff people who seem to be in the most danger of being assaulted are large, young men.

In addition, just like anyone else, clients respond very negatively if a staff person is bossy, controlling, insulting, demanding, or acts very superior. Clients on illegal drugs, such as methamphetamines, can also be unpredictable and dangerous at times, until the drugs get out of their system.

Ambulatory Restraints

"Straight-jackets" as seen in old movies, are no longer used. Clients who continue to be assaultive may be required to wear a device called PADS (personal assault device system.) This consists of a belt around the waist and wrist restraints that control hand movement. The range of the wrist restraints can be adjusted from a few inches to about a foot. But wearing PADS, the person then is allowed to come out of his/her room. In some cases, a similar device is worn on the feet (shackles).

PADS or shackles are very seldom used today. (However, when people are taken to court, they may be required to wear PADS and/or shackles.) The trend is toward using medications instead of physical restraints.

Bed Restraints

Today, clients in Mental Health Units are *rarely restrained in bed*. In years past, physical restraints were used much more often. Each time restraints are used, a full report must be made. Physical restraints can be dangerous to clients. For example, the person may twist around and choke.

Today, the client must be *very dangerous to him/herself or others* in order to be restrained in bed. Sometimes, it might be a medical emergency, such as the client who keeps pulling out a necessary IV or catheter. But, bed restraints are almost a thing of the past in many Mental Health Units.

Safety Precautions for Staff

Doctors and nurses are told to avoid wearing items such as ponytails or long hair, dangling earrings, neckties, or non-breakaway nametag lanyards, for their personal safety.

I remember one doctor who did not listen to us and was wearing a regular (not clip-on) necktie. A client grabbed the tie and the doctor had to be rescued by staff.

Often in addition, if a client becomes threatening, other clients may step in and try to assist. One day, a woman was yelling at me and another client said, "Don't yell at Grandma!" (Many of our clients were raised by their grandmas.)

Self-Defense Classes

All staff people on the Mental Health Units are required to take self-defense classes. In these classes, nurses and other staff learn how to break various holds and other ways to deal with an assaultive client. I never had to use these procedures when I worked on the units. But, it is good to know you have the skills, if needed. (I also wouldn't hesitate to use these procedures if I were attacked on the street.)

The emphasis in the hospital today is on preventing assaults before they occur. *Assault situations are very rare.* Staff members are trained to recognize potential physical acting out before it occurs. Then, *interventional steps can be taken to prevent an outburst.* I repeat, *clients are very rarely assaultive toward staff.* They usually realize we are trying to help them.

ECT: Electro Convulsive Therapy

Years ago, "shock treatments" were quite barbaric. (Chapter 2)

The procedure has greatly improved and is widely used today. The person is pre-medicated. An electric shock is administered, to induce a seizure. The seizure is limited to only one limb, where it can be observed. ECT is done in the Post-Anesthesia Recovery Room (PAR), with all the staff and equipment needed in case of emergency, readily available. ECT has proven very helpful for many people. A special outpatient department within the Mental Health Department at HHC handles the pre- and post-procedure care for people on intermittent maintenance ECT.

Vermin

Occasionally, clients come into the hospital with lice on the body or bedbugs in their clothing. When they come through the Crisis Center, they are showered and given clean clothing. This mostly prevents spread onto the Inpatient Units. However one day, a person was admitted with a large black plastic bag. She had been carefully treated for lice in the Crisis Center. The bag was tightly sealed in the Crisis Center and marked, "DO NOT OPEN!"

The client asked the Mental Health Worker for her bathrobe, which was in the bag. The worker was just about to open the bag when I caught him. If the worker had opened the bag, the lice could have been spread throughout the unit. Good thing I caught him! Occasionally, we needed to treat a client for lice. This was done with special shampoo and a very fine-toothed comb. We prevented mass outbreaks.

SPECIAL STORIES

There are so many stories from my nearly twenty-six years working in the Psychiatry Department at HCMC, I could not begin to tell them all. Following is a sampling:

The Purse Snatcher

One day, one of the older female nurses went outside to put money in her parking meter. She was very thin and probably looked vulnerable and helpless. A man grabbed her purse. She responded automatically, grabbed her purse back, and flipped the man to the ground. I'll bet he was really surprised. That's what he gets for messing with a Psych nurse!

The Foosball Table

We had a huge man, Roberto S, who came in fairly frequently, so we all knew him. He was about six-foot-four and weighed over 350 pounds. (I am five feet tall.) Roberto had been a professional football player and was still in pretty good shape. He was not usually assaultive, but he certainly was large.

One day, I was the only staff for a short time on one of the ICUs. Suddenly, Roberto picked up the large foosball table and held it up over his head. He was yelling at me and threatening to hit me with the heavy table. I could not think of anything else to do.

So, in my loudest "motherly" tone, I said, "*You put that down right now!*" And, he did. I have no idea what I would have done if he had not put it down.

Roberto often "decorated" his hospital room. He used toilet paper and towels and sheets. He was tall enough so he could almost reach the ceiling. The decorating projects kept him busy and he didn't hurt anything.

Roberto's younger brother was also a star football player and was actually more famous than Roberto. He died very young. He was to receive a special award at a football game and Roberto was going to accept it on his behalf. I was at the game and when I saw Roberto later, I told him I had seen him and how proud I was to know him. He just beamed. I am sure he rarely got a compliment. Roberto's brother usually got all the credit and Roberto was left in the shadows.

The Pepper Spray Incident

We had a violent young man who had tried to escape. He was on a court hold. He was very angry and assaultive when he was caught and returned to the unit. He was locked in a "quiet room (Q.R.)" in the ICU for a short time, to allow him to calm down. He was still very agitated, but the guards wanted to try to talk to him.

When the guards opened the door to the quiet room, the client broke the top off a table and was threatening the guards with it. Every time they tried to open the door, he would swing the tabletop at them in a downward chopping motion. And he was also trashing the Q.R. that he was in.

The guards tried everything to get into the room, but were unsuccessful. They really had no alternative but to use pepper spray. They sprayed him once, with no results. They had to spray him several times to get him calmed down enough so they could get into the room and the client could be restrained in his bed. (This needed to be done for everyone's safety.)

The problem with pepper spray is the fumes. This permeated the whole unit. Because the windows only open at the very top, maintenance people had to come with ladders to open them, to get some circulation. By this time, several people (clients and staff) were ill; some were vomiting. None of us had expected this problem. It was really a terrible situation. I have only seen pepper spray used that once. And, I am sure the policy is only to use it for an *extreme life-threatening emergency.*

Police Monitoring and Legal Cases

Sometimes, inmates from jail or prison are admitted to the Mental Health Unit. And, in some cases, they are monitored twenty-four/seven by a police officer. It depends on their crime and the court order. This is very boring for the police officer, because they cannot come onto the unit with a weapon. Usually, one guard sits by the main door and a second one sits in the hall by the back door. We try to stop and talk to them and give them treats occasionally, to help them pass the time.

No Weapons on the Unit

Sometimes, a police officer comes to the unit to meet with a client and refuses to surrender his/her weapon. No one is allowed to have a gun on the unit, to prevent the possibility of a client getting it. There are gun lockers in the sally ports where officers can lock up their guns and keep the key until they are ready to leave. If they are not willing to do this, they have to conduct their business in the sally port, because they cannot come onto the nursing unit.

Threats Against the President

If a person threatens the President or another top government official, the FBI becomes involved. This is a Federal offense and is punishable by law. So, sometimes, we had FBI agents on the units. One man, Spencer B, frequently made threats against the President when he relapsed.

The doctors were able to avoid criminal action against him, because he had such a serious mental illness. He would be allowed to remain in the hospital until he was no longer considered a threat. (This man had the job of putting the Sunday supplements into the newspaper. When you began getting three or four of each supplement or things were otherwise mixed up, we knew we would be getting him back into the hospital soon.)

The Fake Client

We had a young man who was admitted to the hospital saying he was feeling suicidal. He also appeared to be severely mentally challenged. He told us his father had abandoned him at a truck stop and he didn't have anywhere to go. He was very convincing and the staff felt sorry for him. Some even brought him clothes and games. He was allowed to wear street clothes (as did most of the clients in the Mental Health units.)

One day, this young man joined a group of medical students and escaped from the unit by just walking out with them. That very afternoon, the FBI came to our unit, looking for him. We learned that he had a brother who was in fact, mentally challenged, so he had known how to act as though he were disabled. Our client was wanted by the FBI for some serious crime and was using the hospital to hide out. He almost got away with it, but was later caught and prosecuted.

A Car and a Dog

One night close to change of shift at eleven P.M., there was a gunfight in the street near the hospital. We were able to watch it safely from our fifth floor window. We watched the shooting and then watched the police arrest the two men involved. Later, we could see the markers on the sidewalk where bullet casings had fallen.

During this whole event, the entire hospital was locked down for about an hour. Nobody could come in or leave. This included staff and visitors. Some people had difficulty, because they had baby-sitters at home, buses to catch, or rides waiting to pick them up.

When the lockdown was lifted, we were notified that no one could leave without a security or police escort. My escort turned out to be two Minneapolis police officers in a canine unit. Since I was parked in a ramp directly across the street, I had expected them to walk me to my car. I was surprised that they were going to take me in their police car.

The two male officers were in the front seat, so I was instructed to get into the back seat. They had the front seat pushed back so far there was no room for my feet, so I had to put them up on the seat. There was a kind of gate between the front and back seats, so it looked like I was being arrested.

In the back seat, I found myself face to face with a huge police dog, sitting up straight in the seat and staring at me. The officers told me not to pet the dog (which I had no intention of doing.) *This was the dog's seat and he was NOT happy to share it with me.* Every time I moved, even a little, he would glare at me and growl softly under his breath. I doubt if the officers could even hear him.

Even though I was parked just across the street, we had to go around several blocks, because of the one-way streets. Then, the police drove directly into the ramp and right up next to my car. They watched me get in and drive away. It was an interesting experience and I was happy that the dog must have eventually decided I was not a threat.

Two Murderers in the Hospital

The Angry Russian Immigrant and the Grocery Chain Heir

In 1992, two men, Zachary Persitz and Russell Lund, were in the Psych ICU at the same time. They were on the unit called "Orange 8." (This unit was considered the "Forensic Unit," because legal situations were usually handled there.)

The news stories about both men were covered extensively on TV and in newspapers. (Minneapolis Star-Tribune; local TV stations; and Google under Prozumenshikov) Part of the story was also presented in the TV series, "Forensic Files." (Season 11, Episode 2—The title of this episode is "Going for Broke.")

In addition, a book has been written about the story—(The PRU-BACHE MURDER. (See Bibliography) So, *I am not violating anyone's confidentiality.*

Both Zachary and Russell were admitted to the hospital under aliases. (This occurs in high profile cases to provide privacy, reduce publicity, and keep news people away.) Their actual names were used in all the news stories, however.

Zachary

Zachary was admitted from the Hennepin County Jail, because he said he was suicidal. He was admitted to the hospital under the alias of David Hammerstein. He had invested his life savings and also some settlement money from an accident (more than $250,000) with a stockbroker, Michael Prozumenshikov. Zachary trusted Michael, because both were Russian immigrants. The two families were friends and often did things together.

Michael, the stockbroker, lived in a lavish home in a Western Minneapolis suburb and drove a fancy car. However, Zachary's investments had been rapidly losing money, partly as a result of the stock market downturn. In addition, Zachary felt Michael was not handling his investments properly.

It was later learned that Zachary was correct; Michael was making repeated investments in order to make more money. Zachary was threatened with bankruptcy and home foreclosure and blamed Michael for his losses.

On January 28, 1991, Zachary called Michael and demanded a large refund or a promissory note (for $200,000) that same night. Michael was not able to get the items that fast.

To make a long story short, Michael's fancy Mercedes was found abandoned in Wayzata, Minnesota. Later, his headless and dismembered body was found in a dumpsite in another county. (His entire body was never found. However, one finger was with the body and was used to identify him.)

Michael was thirty-seven years old.

Zachary was eventually arrested for the murder; partly because a single hair from a rare breed of dog, a Bernese Mountain Dog, was found with Michael's body and Zachary had one of these dogs. A bumper fragment and paint from Zachary's car was also found at the dumpsite, because Zachary had crashed through the gate to get in.

After a time, Zachary confessed to killing Michael, saying he had "cut him up to prevent identification" and "to keep Michael from haunting him." But before this confession, Zachary fought conviction by pleading "not guilty by reason of insanity." He was in our hospital's Forensic Unit, because he was depressed and also to determine if he was "mentally competent to stand trial."

Russell

Russell was the wealthy heir to a large grocery chain. One day his estranged wife, a former beauty queen, and her "boy friend" came over to discuss divorce plans. Russell killed them both in cold blood. He was arrested almost immediately. This murder was also widely covered in the news. Russell was hospitalized in our Forensic Unit with depression at the same time as was Zachary.

I was working in the Psych ICU at the time and got to know both men quite well.

The Suicide Pact

While they were on our Forensic Unit, Russell and Zachary became friends and made a suicide pact (that they would both commit suicide, using plastic bags.)

Russell's family found out and had him immediately transferred out of our hospital, the county hospital, into a private hospital. He had been on a twenty-four-hour suicide watch at HCMC. But, after he was transferred, he had more freedom and was able to take his life at the second hospital.

Zachary appealed his conviction, but this was denied. He was deemed competent to stand trial and was convicted of murder. He was incarcerated in the Stillwater (Minnesota) prison and also at Oak Park Heights, where he was serving a life sentence for the crime. He would have been eligible to apply for parole in 2021. But, while in prison, he too committed suicide in 2010 by hanging himself. (Star Tribune, April 1, 2015)

He was then fifty-nine years old.

I have a large file of newspaper clippings and articles regarding these two cases. I had planned someday to write a "true crime" book about them. But, I have not done this.

The Nursing Supervisor

One night, a *new young female Nursing Supervisor* came up to our unit where the two murderers were. I had never seen her before. She asked why the two men were admitted using aliases. We explained that high profile cases were often admitted using aliases and that these were the two men who had committed murders and who had been covered so extensively in the news.

Then, one of the people I was working with asked, "Did they ever find that one guy's head?" And we said, "No."

The young, innocent supervisor asked, "You guys are kidding. Right?" And we said, "No." She left the unit quickly and *we never saw her again*. She either quit, or refused to ever come back to Psych!

MORE FAVORITE STORIES

The Catheterization

When I first started on Psych, I had to do a urinary catheterization on a woman client. Her legs were severely contracted and it was difficult to perform the procedure. In addition, I had not done one for a number of years. I did it and it went okay. Then, I told our unit Instructor about it and at first she said, "You should have had me help you." Then, she said, "But I'm really glad you didn't, because I haven't done one for many years."

Two Fires

One day, I was talking to a client named Bob. He said, "I can't understand why I got evicted from my apartment. *It was just a little fire.*" It turns out that he had not paid his gas and electric bills, so he was cooking (inside his apartment) on a charcoal grill. The curtains caught fire, but as he said, "It was just a little fire." However, the landlord didn't agree with him.

A relative of mine was married to a woman who had bipolar Illness ("manic depression.") Sometimes, she was very manic. When this occurred, she wrote and wrote, day and night. While she was writing, she burned many candles. One time, the curtains in their home caught fire and when her husband came home, he was barely able to save her and their children.

The Bathroom Fight

I was working night shift and in the middle of the night I heard loud yelling in one of the four-bed men's wards. I went in to see what was going on. One of the men had gotten up to go to the bathroom. He didn't turn on the light and sat down on the toilet. Another man also got up and went into the bathroom without turning on the light. He began urinating while the first man was sitting on the toilet. Of course, the man who was sitting got all wet.

It was very hard for me not to laugh. Eventually, the men realized it was funny, took showers, and went back to bed.

But, for a short time, I had to be a *referee*. Nurses have many functions.

My Limited Spanish

I only speak a little Spanish, having taken Spanish years ago in college. One day, working on the *eighth floor* at night, I was talking to a man who spoke no English. This man refused to sleep in his bed, so he slept on the couch in the lounge. When I questioned him he said, "There is a man outside my window and he scares me and it makes my testicles hot." (Now, it is important to remember that even if you speak a little of a foreign language, it is very difficult to understand if it doesn't make sense.)

When I documented the encounter, I wrote that *this was what I thought he had said*. The next day, we had a Spanish-speaking doctor on the unit and I asked her to find out if that was what he actually had said. She talked to him and indeed, my interpretation was correct. She was also able to explain to him that he was not in any danger since he was on the eighth floor and he began sleeping in his bed.

Interpreters

The hospital now has a system for interpreting almost any language. The last I heard, we had facilities to interpret over fifty languages. Some of this is done in person by Certified Interpreters and some is done by telephone or Internet. This makes hospitalization much more comfortable and safe for foreign clients (and their staff.) Many staff members are also multilingual, although they are not Certified Interpreters.

The Missing Door

One day, one of the clients damaged their bathroom door. So, the door was removed and placed in a storage room at the end of the hall. The entrance to this room went in a couple of feet to a wall and then turned to the left. The door was propped up against the wall, directly in front of the entrance.

The Maintenance Man came to repair the door and asked where it was. I told him. He came back in a few minutes and said, "I can't find any door in that room." I wondered if someone had moved the door, so I went down to the storeroom with him.

Of course, the door was right in front of his nose where I said it was. I took him by the hand, pointed to the door and said, "Door!" He said, "Don't tell my wife. She says I can't find anything." (I guess this could be called "*male-pattern blindness*" which afflicts many men, including my husband.)

Trip to Viet Nam

We had a man who was suffering from PTSD/PTS (post-traumatic stress/disorder.) One day, I walked by him as he was talking to a very young female peer. She must have asked him why he was in the hospital and I heard him say, "Well, I was in Viet Nam in the '60s." And, she exclaimed, "*Oh, on vacation?*" I nearly fainted. (And, the young woman had absolutely *no clue* about the war in Viet Nam.)

The Viet Nam Missionary

As an aside, when I was a nursing student, the Viet Nam war had not yet begun. One of my nursing classmates, Vurnell, was planning to go to Viet Nam as a medical missionary after graduation. None of us had ever heard of Viet Nam at that time, so we had to look it up on a map. Our classmate and her husband did go there.

Unfortunately, her husband was murdered by the Viet Cong. She stayed in Viet Nam and married again. They stayed in Viet Nam for a number of years, working for Wycliffe Bible Translators. She is now working for Wycliffe in the U.S. at the age of eighty-plus.

Wash Your Hands

We had a man who masturbated constantly in his room. He came to the desk one day and said he wanted to go make a sandwich. The nurse I was working with said with a straight face, *"Be sure you wash your hands first."*

The Nursing Strike

There was a nursing strike in Minneapolis in 2016. HCMC was not on strike, because we were considered a "safety net hospital," furnishing emergency care for the Southern part of Hennepin County. Many nurses were brought in from other parts of the country to care for hospital patients in the absence of the striking nurses. One evening, there was a news story on TV about the strike and it showed some of the replacement nurses. One was walking down the street wearing hospital scrubs. However on closer inspection, she was wearing about three-inch high heels. I wonder how difficult it would be to do nursing care in those shoes?

The Space Ship

The Hubert H. Humphrey Metrodome football stadium was just across the street, easily visible from the windows of some of the Psych units.

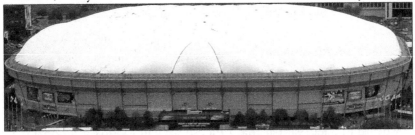

Hubert H. Humphrey Metrodome, Minneapolis, Minnesota (Wikimedia)

It was round with a special fabric top. It had lights around the edges. It did in fact, look a lot like a space ship.

One of our clients had a fixed delusion about the stadium. She was convinced it was a space ship and that it had brought her into Minneapolis from her planet. She was anxious to get out of the hospital, so she could catch the ship to go back to her home. She was particularly delusional about the stadium at night, when the lights around the stadium were on. We tried, to no avail, to convince her that it was a football stadium and not a space ship.

However, this whole situation became a much greater problem when the stadium was torn down, to make way for the new Minnesota Vikings stadium. Then, she was convinced that the space ship had left without her.

Pets

It was always refreshing to have pets brought up to the unit. Sometimes, the Humane Society would bring animals to visit. Sometimes staff people and visitors had animals that had been specially trained and certified as helper dogs or cats.

We sometimes had clients who did not talk to anyone. But, when they saw an animal, they talked and cooed to the animal. It was so sweet to see. And, it was very helpful to the clients (and to the staff.)

One of the units had a resident rabbit for a long time. It finally became too much trouble for the staff to care for the rabbit on the unit, so he went to live with one of them full time.

The Shopping Trip

One day, a friend from my hometown was in Minneapolis. We decided to go to a thrift store, which at that time was on Hennepin Avenue, next to a soup kitchen. Since it was lunchtime, there was a long line of people, mostly men, waiting to get in to eat their meal.

As it happened, I knew many of them from the hospital. My friend, being from a small town was shocked. She was a nurse and had graduated from a private school, but she had not met homeless people before. Her eyes got bigger and bigger as we walked down the street and all the people greeted me. I didn't think anything of it, because I knew these people.

The Pregnancy Test

I was admitting a forty-two-year-old woman to the Psych unit. Pregnancy tests are often done because psych medications can be very toxic to a developing fetus. So, I asked her if there was any possibility that she could be pregnant. She replied, "No, but I masturbate a lot."

Interesting Clients

Elvis Reborn

We had a young man who was born on the actual day Elvis Presley died. He was convinced that he was Elvis reborn. He had the hair-do, wore the clothes, and practiced singing like Elvis. He really was very convincing and his singing was very good. I think he actually did some Elvis impersonations around the Twin Cities when he was doing better. However, the Elvis delusion remained a permanent part of his personality.

The Courtship/Wedding

We had a man named Kurt who was totally convinced he was dating a certain woman. He would call her at all hours of the day and night. He stalked her by sitting outside her home. I knew her too and she was not interested in him and wanted nothing to do with him. In fact, she was afraid of him.

She could not get him to leave her alone. Unfortunately, she eventually felt she had to move out of state and change her name to get away from him. This went on for a number of years. One time I saw him and he told me all about this girl friend. Then, the next time I saw him, he told me they were engaged. Then, he told me they had gotten married. Next, they had a baby. This delusion went on until Kurt died when he was only in his early 40s.

The Banana Phone

We had a lady who walked around the unit all day holding a banana to her ear and talking to it as though it were a phone. One day, she forgot and ate her banana. When she realized what she had done, she was hysterical. "Now I can't make any calls!" We had to search the entire hospital to find another banana for her. And, then everything was okay.

Hoarder Homes

We often admitted people who lived in trash houses. (Chapter 3) These were like the places you see on the "Hoarder" TV programs. This is a true illness. The police often brought photos of these homes when they brought clients in.

In many cases, there was not even a path; the person had to climb over stuff to move around the home. Usually, the kitchen was no longer usable. Often, the bathroom was non-functioning as well. In many cases, the person was not able to sleep in a bed.

In extreme hoarding like this, it is not only a health and fire hazard, but if the person became physically ill or injured, rescue people would not be able to evacuate them.

We admitted a woman who had fifty-seven cats and lived in a trash house. Of course, the cats were inbred and some of them were sick, but she loved them all. One day, I was talking to her and she said, "They are only going to let me keep six cats when I get out. I feel really bad." (I was surprised they were going to let her keep that many.)

Another hoarder person had two cats. He died suddenly. Workers were feeding the cats, but they never saw them. There were so many places for the cats to hide that it took several weeks to find them, after everything was cleaned out. The cats were just fine, but they were afraid.

Super Glue

A young woman used Super Glue to glue her vaginal labia together (twice). In this case, surgery was required in order to allow her to urinate.

The Bariatric Woman

We had a woman who weighed 530 pounds. She had been brought in by ambulance. I was assigned to discharge her with her friend who had a van. I called the hospital transportation people and they said their largest wheelchair was rated at a maximum of 550 pounds. So, they sent the wheelchair and four people to assist.

We were not able to get the woman into the van because she could not step up the eight or so inches to get into the van and we could not lift her. So, she had to be transported back to her home by ambulance. I friend of mine knows her and says she has gained even more weight since her discharge from the hospital. She is totally immobile now.

"So, I Had to Kill Him!"

We admitted a lady from jail. I knew she was charged with felony murder. When I was talking to her, she was explaining her situation.

She calmly told her story this way: "I was married to this guy and he beat me up. I divorced him and married another guy. And, the second guy started to beat me up. I told him I was not going to go through that again and he'd better stop or else. He beat me again, so I had to kill him." This was said very matter-of-factly, without the slightest emotion. But, you have to admit, she did warn him ahead of time. I really wondered about the truthfulness of her story, but it was, in fact, true.

Sexual Reassignment Stories

We have had a number of people over the years undergoing sexual reassignment. Most often, these are men transitioning to women. Sometimes, they complete the process, but not always. They may come into the hospital for counseling during the process or if they change their minds or become indecisive about it. Treatment procedures have changed greatly over the years.

The Pink Nightgown

Years ago, we had a very large and tall man who was a farm worker. He was in the process of becoming a woman. At that time, the process was very rare and these clients did not have private rooms. This man was in a four-bed ward with three other men. During the day, he wore bib overalls. At night, he wore a long pink flannel nightgown and pink rollers in his hair. And, none of his roommates ever complained. I have no idea if he completed the process or not. Today any person having gender reassignment in housed in a private room.

"I've Decided to be a Boy"

I met a young man in downtown Minneapolis one day. He looked familiar, but I couldn't place him, although I knew he was from the hospital. He rushed up to me and greeted me excitedly. Then he said, "I have to tell you. I went to college, I've got a good job, I have a nice apartment, and I've decided to be a boy!" This was all in one sentence.

It was then that I remembered the last time I had seen him. He was in the process of undergoing the medical and surgical processes required to become a female. He had been wearing a woman's hairdo, dressing in female clothing, and using a female name. It was wonderful to see him and great to know he was doing so well and that he had made a final decision about his sexuality.

My Relatives

I had a relative who had five sons. Many years ago, the two oldest sons had sexual reassignment surgery. I think they went to Sweden, because this procedure was not yet done in this country. Their father could never accept this fact and basically disowned his two boys, who were now girls. It was very sad and was a closely guarded secret among my relatives. Everyone in the family denied it or pretended it hadn't happened. It was as though these two boys had never existed. I have no idea where they are now.

PERSONAL STORIES

My Friend's Daughter

One of my best friends had a daughter, Marie G, who had very serious mental health issues. She came into HCMC from time to time. One day, she was on a unit downstairs and I got a call. They asked if I knew her and I said I did. They said she was totally out of control, screaming and demanding to see "Caroline." I went down and talked to her and then everything was fine. She just needed a little reassurance from someone she knew.

Jack and "Caroline Bunker"

My maiden name was Bunker. Jack S, a man I had known in college, was admitted. He had severe mental health issues. I did not realize he was on my unit until I got into shift-change report and then it was too late for me to change units. So, I went to Jack and told him I would not be reading his chart or looking at any of his personal information.

He said, "Caroline Bunker can read my chart any time."

One of the other nurses overheard this and said, "You really have known him for a long time!"

My last name had been Rosdahl for more than fifty years. (Jack died in 2018 at the age of seventy-nine.)

The First Computers in the Hospital

We got computers in the hospital in the early 2000s.

My supervisor John Gray, came to me and said, "We are getting computers, but we will help you."

I was quite familiar with word processing, since I had been writing books for years.

As it happened, I was about the only nurse who even knew how to turn a computer on. So, after a few days, John came to me again and said, "Could you help the others figure out the computers?"

After that, many younger nurses were hired and they were all familiar with computer use.

More recently, when many of the nurses were young, all the computers went out. All the nurses just stood there and didn't know what to do. I said, "Get a piece of paper and a pencil and go talk to one of the clients."

By that time, the nurses had become dependent on the computers. (And, in all honesty, some functions could not be performed without them.)

The CPR Class

I had to take my biennial CPR class at the age of eighty. The instructor came up to me and asked if I could get down on the floor. I said, "*Yes, I can get down. But, I'm not sure if I can get up again!*" But, I did.

"BOO!!"

It was mid-winter and I was on my way to the morning shift at six-thirty A.M. It was pitch dark. Suddenly, a young man jumped out of a doorway and yelled, "BOO!" As it turned out he had been one of our Psych clients, so I knew him. Otherwise, I would have been really scared. I asked him not to do that again, because he could really scare someone, and he agreed.

Warren

We had a client named Warren S. He walked with a severe limp and often dressed in very unusual ways. One day, I was walking down the street in Downtown Minneapolis with my son Keith, and we met Warren. He had several towels wrapped around his head and was wearing a hospital bathrobe on top of his winter jacket. We talked for a few minutes and Warren continued on down the street. And then, Keith said, "I'll bet I know where you know him from."

Impact on Clients

As a nurse, you usually don't know the impact you make on patients/clients. I am including a note I received from a young man many years ago. I have not seen him since. I believe he has remained well and safe. I hope so.

"*I just want you to know that you have changed my life. I am sure I will never be in a Psych hospital again, but I will never forget you and what you have done for me. Thank you.*" (Justin, 1998)

Survival

Many people do whatever they have to do in order to survive.

The Cowboy Boots

For example, I remember the man who was badly beaten and brought into the hospital. He laughed and said, "Ha, ha. They didn't get my money." He had hollowed out the heels of his cowboy boots and had several thousand dollars hidden there.

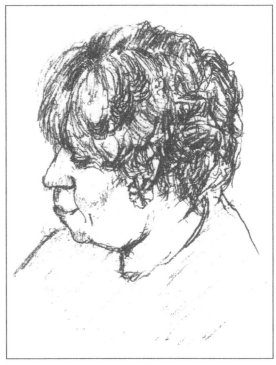

"My Nurse, Caroline," drawn by a client (J Y, 2000, BH Media)

The Itinerant Dog

We admitted a lady who had been traveling all over the country on the bus. She had two duffel bags and she had a little dog, which had been living in the bags. Of course, she could not always let the dog out to go to the bathroom, so the bags were full of dog feces, as well as her belongings. She was admitted to the hospital and one of the women in the Crisis Center took the dog home to care for it.

I was assigned to admit this lady, which involved listing her property. She had a number of magazines in her bags, covered with dog feces. And, throughout the magazines, she had stashed money. Hundreds of dollars.

I counted the money, entered it on her property sheet, and put it in a plastic bag, according to policy.

I took the bag down to the vault and handed it to the lady there. I said, "There is $1,745.00 in this bag."

She said, with a sneer, "Well, you know I have to count it."
I said, "Go ahead."
She opened the bag, took one sniff and said, "I guess I'll take your word for it!"

The Bottom Line

It is important to remember that people with psychiatric issues are more like us than they are unlike us. They have dreams and hopes. They want to make plans. Often, they do very well in the community. Many people are very talented. They are musicians, artists, poets, and writers. I have a large collection of items that have been given to me by my clients.

In some cases, it is sad, because the illness can be progressive. These are the sad stories, but many of the stories are very hopeful. Many clients come into the hospital and we never see them again.

One young man, Herbert A, was brilliant. He wrote very insightful poems and stories. But, one day he said to me, "I used to have a life. I had a job. Now, I am failing. I am just struggling to keep going."

SCHIZOPHRENIA
I am a difficult person, I get obstreperous,
I break things. I raise my voice over imagined insults.
I'm unemployable. What good am I?
Would you invite me into our house?
It's a field day for naysayers.
And, it makes naysayers out of good folk.
It leaves me defenseless.
At the mercy of the court.
As much as anyone else,
As an angry young man,
I would give the finger,
But now I just linger.
Too long, at 48!
(Herbert, 2008)

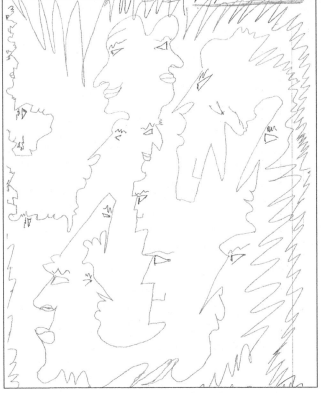

"Schizophrenia", drawn by a client (Charles, 1998, BH Media)

Famous Last Words: "Quotable Quotes" of clients:

- "I just sit home and listen to music, smoke my crack, and read my Bible." (Calvin)

- "I'm the great harlot; I'm the antichrist." (Connie)

- "My mental status has nothing to do with my mental illness." (Marjorie)

- "The street lights told me to do it" (to steal cars.) (Norman)

- "You will be my Number One Assistant when I go to Heaven." (Bob)

Selected Works of Mental Health Clients
(All these items are used with permission of the authors.)

CAROLINE
C Caring,
A Always
R Returning,
O Only to
L Love some more,
I Individually,
N Natural,
E Each and every day.
(Barbara, 1995)

PANIC
Closer, creeping,
Never showing its fully wicked self.
I can feel the overflowing fear,
With no one to help.
I've seen the black wall of panic,
Quickly falling towards me.
Never really leaving, Cut short breathing,
Making me believe that I'll never be free.
Those who supposedly understand, but haven't been there,
Are ignorant and don't know despair.
If you want to know what it's like, just try to see,
An invisible, unbeatable night.
It seems it's going away sometimes,
Or is it I'm just getting used to it?
But, the ugly head rears, and I say to myself,
Don't ever give up and never ever quit.
(David, 2003)

MORNING GLORY
Morning Glory—that is what she called me one day.
"Are you talking to me?" I asked.
"Yes", she retorted. And, then her face relaxed.
"I have never been called names like that before." I said, trying
*   to hold back the tears of joy.*
"Well, you had better get used to it", she said, with that delight-
*   ful smile on her face.*
"Why Mother, why would you call me names like morning glory
*   in the first place?"*
"Because, my lovely child, you bring me so much happiness."
"Well, there is something I would like to say if I may."
"Thank you, my friend, my mentor, and my new mother,
For making me feel this special of a daughter."
"To Caroline. Wishing you all the best. Thank you for being my
*   new mother."*
From a patient—(Debbie, 1999)

The Community Advisory Committee

In the past year, I have been appointed as a member of the Community Advisory Committee to the Department of Psychiatry at the University of Minnesota. One of the situations we are addressing is homelessness among people with mental health challenges. In addition, the committee is concerned about improving the public's image of mental illness. A yearly symposium attracts attendees from community agencies, as well as educators from several states. I am honored to be on this committee.

FINAL STORIES

The Admission Questionnaire

This is one of my favorite nursing stories of all time.

I was admitting a lady to the hospital and asking all the routine questions—

"When was your last menstrual period?

"When was your last bowel movement?

"Are you feeling threatened at home?"

When I asked her the next question on the list, "Are you sexually active?" she looked around and then looked thoughtfully at the ceiling for several seconds.

She then replied, in all seriousness, "No, I pretty much just lie there!"

The Psych Client Who Thought He Could Fly

I will end this book by repeating the reason for the book's title.

When I was working at the County Hospital in the 1960s, late one very cold winter night a male Psych client demanded to leave. Since he was on a hold, he could not legally be discharged from the hospital. I explained this to him and the next thing I saw was him running down the length of the ward with me right behind him.

He smashed through the window of the third- floor porch at a dead run and never missed a beat, as he landed in a bush and a snowbank, and took off running down 7th Street in Minneapolis.

I called the police and they asked, "Is there any way we could recognize him?" I said "Well, he is probably the only man running down 7th Street in an open-backed hospital gown and paper slippers."

It didn't take long for them to locate him and bring him back to the hospital!

There are many stories in "The Naked City!"

The clients are very serious about what they say. You can't laugh at them. And, *I could never make up this stuff.*

And, the stories go on and on and on.

Nursing is always an ongoing and unpredictable adventure.

APPENDIX A

AUTHOR'S EDUCATION
AND LICENSURE

CAROLINE BUNKER ROSDAHL, RN-BC, ALA, BSN, PHN, MA
Registered Nurse

Board Certified by American Nurses' Credentialing Center (ANCC)

Associate in Liberal Arts Degree

Bachelor of Science in Nursing

Certified Public Health Nurse

Certified School Nurse (K-12)

Master of Arts—Education and Psychology

ABT (All, but Thesis), PhD, University of Minnesota

Life Certificate—K-12 School Counselor

Basic Life Support Certificate

MN Certified Vocational Teacher Educator

APPENDIX B

SELECTED HONORS AND AWARDS IN NURSING AND EDUCATION

Recipient: Distinguished Alumnus (1 of 100, a one-time event), University of Minnesota School of Nursing, Centennial Celebration, 2009

Recipient: Verna Mae Blomquist Award for Excellence in Vocational Education, 1969

Teacher of the Year, Delta Kappa Gamma Society for Women Educators, 1970

Named in "Worldwide Leaders in HealthCare", International Nurses' Association, 2016, 2017

Listed in "Who's Who in the Midwest": 1994-1995

Named in: "Who's Who in American Nursing": 1993-1994, 1996-1997

"Director's Friend" Award: University of Minnesota Bands, 1992

National Honor Society, Sauk Centre High School, 1953-1955

National Advisory Committee, High School Health Careers, McGraw-Hill, New York, 1976-1978

Presidents' Award, Minnesota Technical Institute Assistant Directors' Association, 1987-1988

PROFESSIONAL ASSOCIATIONS

Current Member—Community Advisory Committee, Department of Psychiatry, University of Minnesota, 1917 to Present

Current Board Member and Former President—Board of Directors, University of Minnesota Band Alumni Society

Minnesota and American MENSA

Member: Sigma Theta Tau, Honor Society in Nursing, Zeta Chapter, 1984

Current Member, Delta Kappa Gamma, International Society for Women in Education

Former Member—Alumni Board, College of Education, University of Minnesota

Former Member—Alumni Board, School of Nursing, University of Minnesota

Former Liaison to the School of Nursing Foundation Board

Former Member, Society of Manufacturing Engineers

APPENDIX C

PUBLICATIONS
BY CAROLINE ROSDAHL

Author: TEXTBOOK OF BASIC NURSING (Editions 2-11), Lippincott/ WoltersKluwer, Philadelphia, now in its 11ᵗʰ Edition (2017—"50ᵗʰ Anniversary Edition"), plus Indonesian translation in 5 volumes

Consultant and Editor: Nursing and Allied Health Series (7 books), McGraw-Hill, New York, 1976-1978; (Chapter 12) Titles include:

YOUR CAREER IN HEALTH CARE, by Beverly Rambo and Diane Watson, 1976.

BASIC SCIENCES FOR HEALTH CAREERS, by Karl Wittman, 1976.

INTRODUCTION TO NURSING CARE, by R. Winifred Johnson and Douglass Johnson, 1976, (a Nursing Assistant text.)

PRINCIPLES AND PRACTICE OF NURSING CARE by Donna Story, 1976, (a beginning practical nursing text.)

WORKBOOK to accompany PRINCIPLES AND PRACTICE, by Donna Story, 1976.

MEDICAL LABORATORY SKILLS, by Karl Wittman and John Thomas, 1977.

WARD CLERK SKILLS, by Beverly Rambo, 1978.

Author: Chapter 6, *"Ages and Stages, the Ever-Changing Child"* in HOME-MAKING FOR TEEN-AGERS, Ed 3, Bennett Books, (Pages 66-125), Peoria IL, 1972. (Chapter 12)

 CORNEAL SURGERY: Theory, Technique, and Tissue, Ed. 2. Edited by Frederick S. Brightbill, Mosby, St. Louis, 1993. In Chapter 52, *"Shared Services for Procuring Tissues and Organs"*, Pages 725- 733. (Chapter 12)

Contributor to Davis' NCLEX PN Review by Patricia Beare, 1994.

Consultant to an exploratory book for younger children: THE HOSPITAL—Doctors, Nurses, and Mystery Workers, by Carolyn London, 1976.

Plus several Journal Articles and miscellaneous other publications.

Article about Rosdahl: "*She Wrote the Book*" in MINNESOTA NURSE, May 16, 1994, Page 7.

Editor-in-Chief: MAINSTREETER, the school newspaper for Sauk Centre High School, 1954-1955.

APPENDIX D

AUTHOR'S PERTINENT EMPLOYMENT EXPERIENCES

Staff Nurse, Hennepin County Medical Center, Minneapolis MN

Vice-President Emeritus, Anoka Technical College, Anoka MN

Director, Practical Nursing Program, Anoka Technical College

Director, Wright County Public Health Nursing Service, Buffalo MN

Executive Director, Minnesota Lions' Eye Bank, University of Minnesota

School Nurse/Counselor, Hopkins High School, Hopkins MN

Staff Nurse/Float Pool, Minneapolis General Hospital, Minneapolis MN

Triage and Referral Nurse, National Insurance Company, Eden Prairie MN

Case Manager, Abbott-Northwestern Home Care, Minneapolis MN

Nursing Assistant, St. Michael's Hospital, Sauk Centre MN

Instructor at all levels of Nursing, including: Nursing Assistant, Practical Nursing, 2-year Associate Degree Nursing Program, 3-year Diploma Nursing Program, and 4-year Baccalaureate Nursing Program

OTHER EMPLOYMENT:

Clerk, Grossman's Variety Store, Sauk Centre MN

Interviewer, Burke Marketing Research, Cincinnati OH

Owner/Operator, Dairy Queen, Buffalo MN

Helper, LaPorte (Minnesota) Cream Station

BIBLIOGRAPHY

Adams-Ender, Brigadier General (Ret.) Clara (with Blair Walker.) MY RISE TO THE STARS . . . *How a Sharecropper's Daughter Became an Army General.* Lake Ridge VA, Cape Associates, 2001.

Barnard, Christiaan (studied under Wangensteen). ONE LIFE, New York City, Macmillan, 1969.

Buchwald, Henry, MD. SURGICAL RENAISSANCE IN THE HEART-LAND . . . *a Memoir of the Wangensteen Era.* Minneapolis MN, University of Minnesota Press, 2020.

Carlson, Gretchen. BE FIERCE . . . *Stop Harassment and Take Your Power Back.* Hachette Group, Center Street, 2017.

Carlson, Gretchen. GETTING REAL. Penguin (Random House), 2015.

Compton, Ida L. SINCLAIR LEWIS AT THORVALE FARM . . . *A Personal Memoir.* Compton Estate, 1988.

Egan, Jennifer. MANHATTAN BEACH. New York NY, Scribner, 2017.

Engel, Leonard. THE OPERATION . . . *a minute-by-minute account of a heart operation---and the story of medicine and surgery that led up to it.* New York NY, McGraw-Hill, 1958.

Glass, Laurie K. LEADING THE WAY . . . *the University of Minnesota School of Nursing*—1909-2009. Tasora Books, 2010.

Gray, James. EDUCATION FOR NURSING . . . *a History of the University of Minnesota School.* University of Minnesota Press, 1960.

Hamilton, Lynn. FLORENCE NIGHTINGALE . . . *a Life Inspired.* Wyatt North, Kindle Store eBook, Amazon.com.

Herbert, Raymond, PhD. Florence Nightingale: *Saint, Reformer, or Rebel.* Malabar FL, Robert Krieger Publishing, 1981.

Koblas, John. SINCLAIR LEWIS—HOME AT LAST. Bloomington MN, Voyageur Press, 1981.

Krugerud, Mary (Editor). THE GIRL IN BUILDING C . . . *the True Story of a Teenage Tuberculosis Patient.* Minnesota Historical Society Press, 2018.

Lewis, Sinclair. ARROWSMITH . . . *The Story of Doc Vickerson and an Epidemic.* New York NY, Harcourt, Brace and Company, 1925. (There are many other books by Lewis.)

Lewis, Sinclair. MAIN STREET . . . the Story of Carol Kennicott. New York NY, Harcourt, Brace and Company, 1920.

Nightingale, Florence. NOTES ON NURSING . . . *What it is and What it is not.* (Nightingale's principles for the care of the sick and injured.) With commentaries by contemporary nursing leaders. Philadelphia PA, J.B. Lippincott, Commemorative Edition, 1992. Originally published in 1859. (There are many other books by and about Nightingale.)

Nolan, Jeanette Covert. Florence Nightingale. New York NY, Julian Messner Inc., 1956.

Olson, Roberta. SINCLAIR LEWIS . . . *The Journey.* Sauk Centre MN, Roberta Olson, 1990.

Parry, Sally, Editor. The Minnesota Stories of SINCLAIR LEWIS. St. Paul MN, Borealis Books, Minnesota Historical Society Press, 2005.

Schorer, Mark. SINCLAIR LEWIS . . . *An American Life.* New York NY, McGraw-Hill, 1961.

Taylor, Jeffrey. THE PRU-BACHE MURDER . . . *the Fast Life and Grisly Death of a Millionaire Stockbroker.* New York NY, Harper-Collins, 1984.

Tingley, Al. CORNER ON MAIN STREET . . . *True Stories of the Innkeepers on Sinclair Lewis Avenue.* St. Cloud MN, Creative Concepts, 1984.

Wangensteen, Owen MD and Sarah Wangensteen. THE RISE OF SURGERY *from Empiric Craft to Scientific Discipline* (and many other books and articles.) Folkstone, Kent, Dawson, 1978.

Warner, Phillip. The Crimean War. Taplinger Publishing Co. Inc., 1972.

Watson, Diane. EVALUATING COSTS AND DEMONSTRATING THE VALUE OF REHABILITATION SERVICE. American Occupational Therapy Associates Inc., 2000.

Watson, Diane (and Gregg Landry). TASK ANALYSIS: *an Individual, Group, and Population Approach*. AOTA Press, 2014.

Webb, Val. Florence Nightingale: *The Making of a Radical Theologian*. Chance Press, 2002. (Webb was an Adjunct Professor at the U of Minnesota.)

Woodham-Smith, Mrs. (Blanche) Cecil. Florence Nightingale. New York NY, McGraw-Hill, 1951.

MEDICAL ADVANCEMENTS IN MY LIFETIME

GENERAL CHANGES

- More male nurses, much better salaries for all nurses

- More female doctors

- Nurses of all races and ethnicity; ability to wear traditional ethnic/religious clothing at work

- Computer use widespread; ability to access patient records from a distance; improved monitoring of medications; much medical information available on -line

- More attention given to ethnicity; language translators available, ethnic customs followed

- 9-1-1 system available in most US locations for emergency services

NURSING/MECICAL EDUCATION CHANGESS

- More complex education for all levels of nurses

- Nurse specialists: eg. Nurse Practitioner, Physicians' Assistant

- Changes in delivery of nursing education: simulation, distance learning, self-study, learning at one's own pace, less hands-on clinical experience, clinical specialties included in some nursing programs

- Doctors in several locations can conference regarding a patient

- Continuing education required and readily available for medical personnel

- Physicians more often specialized in area of practice; fewer General Practitioners

- Nurses wear scrub suits, rather than white uniforms, no nurses' caps or school pins worn

HOSPITAL CHANGES/ CHANGES IN DELIVERY OF HEALTH CARE

- Virtual/distance care provided when possible; patients may see non-physician; much care delivered by non-physicians

- Hospital admissions based on severity of illness; fewer overnight stays

- Nearly all single or double rooms; no large wards

- Community clinics available to treat homeless and indigent patients

- Many surgeries performed in Day Surgery; no hospitalization necessary

- Interim rehabilitation care provided, rather than longer hospital stay

- More safety in blood transfusions; ability to use only blood components

- Premature infants often survive; many abnormalities can be determined and treated early; conditions may be treated in utero (before birth)

- Better and earlier care for children with disabilities (mental, emotional, physical, educational)

- Early identification and treatment for special needs (eg: autism, various physical disabilities)

- Psychiatric and Chemical Dependency facilities available for all patients

- Immunizations available for many childhood diseases; new ones constantly being discovered;

- Hundreds of new medications; more broad-spectrum antibiotics; some older medications found to be dangerous and removed from the market

- Many birth control methods now available; abortions now legal in most states

- Much better cancer management; many combinations of chemotherapy agents

- More use of stem cells for treatment

- Much improvement in nursing home care and home care services; provide activities and stimulation

- School Nurse works with a team, including social workers, dentists, physical therapists, and personal caregivers; home visits are common

- Many improvements in Rehabilitation Care and equipment; stand-up walkers, specially-adapted wheelchairs, walk-in bathtubs, circle beds, electronic muscle stimulation (to facilitate movement)

- Hotel swimming pools often have patient lifts, to assist disabled people

- Hospital rooms have patient lifts, piped-in oxygen, wall suction, etc

- Service dogs and other animals trained to assist clients with disabilities, such as poor blood sugar control, seizures, limited vision, and limited mobility

- Physical restraints rarely used in Psychiatry; better understanding and treatment of mental health disorders; many new psychiatric medications; ECT often used for maintenance

- Ships and medical teams go to underserved parts of the world to deliver care

- Genetic studies and DNA testing used to improve care

- Injections given by nurses and pharmacists, as well as physicians

- Many changes in infant delivery: midwife, home delivery, rooming-in

- Breast milk pumped for working mothers to give to baby later

- Helicopter transfer available in many locations

- Greater awareness of physical disabilities; ramps, power doors, adapted automobiles, special parking places, etc.

- More specialized treatment available, eg: Physical Therapy, acupuncture, massage, chiropractic, and other non-traditional methods more accepted by the medical community

- Many new disorders discovered and requiring specialized care (eg: HIV/Aids and other autoimmune disorders)

SURGICAL ADVANCEMENTS

- Huge advancements in surgery (open-heart, heart surgery via blood vessels); tiny incision, eg, stents, heart valve replacements, treatment for patent ductus

- Incision closures done with glue, staples, as well as stitches

- Aability to do many surgeries without major incision ("stab wound"), eg: gall-bladder removal, appendix removal, hysterectomy, stomach stapling and other bariatric procedures, etc.

- Brain surgery often done with patient awake

- Repair of fractures with pins and/or external fixators; joint replacements

- Heart, lung, kidney and other transplants

- Ability to reattach severed limbs

- Ability to repair severed blood vessels, replace blood vessels

- New modalities for tremors, Parkinson's and other brain disorders, eg: Gamma Knife, DBS (Deep Brain Stimulation), ultrasound, etc.

- Microsurgery performed, such as eye surgery (cornea replacement, cataracts, etc.)

- Laser surgery used, especially in eye conditions

- Many advancements in bariatric surgery (stomach sleeve, stomach stapling, etc.)

- 3-D body parts can be artificially manufactured and used

- Sex-change surgeries commonly done

EQUIPMENT CHANGES

- Many patient rooms have cardiac monitors, blood pressure monitors, etc.

- Wrist blood pressure monitors; temporal thermometers available

- Blood sugar levels measured externally

- Insulin pumps implanted, to deliver specific doses of insulin; other medication pumps available, such as for pain control

- Bariatric equipment available for morbidly obese patients: beds, wheelchairs and other special equipment (may have 500 pound llimit)

- Mechanical beds alternate pressure, to prevent bedsores and other deformities

- Beds can tilt to treat shock; beds can be made firm, to allow for CPR

- Hospital beds can weigh patient with the patient in bed

- Mechanical CPR available; AED (Automatic External Defibrillators) available for community emergency use

- Automatic defibrillators can be implanted for clients with chronic cardiac conditions

- Ambulances fully equipped with rescue items; staffed by Paramedics; ability to stand up in ambulance to deliver care

- Seat belts and air bags installed in automobiles; use mandatory in many places

- Hyperbaric chambers available in most locations; fixed system or portable

- Mechanical suction widely used

- Mechanical ventilators available

- IV pumps monitor delivery of IV fluids; IVs mixed by Pharmacy, not nurses

- Many more diagnostic systems available; ultrasound, mammogram, colonoscopy, CT scan, cardiac monitors; improved x-ray procedures for diagnosis and treatment

- Retractable injection needles, to prevent needle sticks

- Most medical supplies used for one patient only and then discarded

- Portable oxygen and oxygen concentrators available, to provide mobility for clients

- Autopsies more definitive in forensic medicine

MEET THE AUTHOR

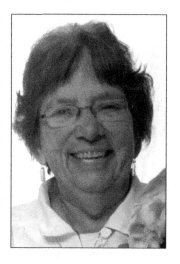

Caroline Bunker Rosdahl has been involved in nursing and health care for nearly seventy years, beginning as a "Nurses' Aide" at age fifteen. She has been involved in many facets of nursing:

She taught nursing at all levels, as well as training nursing assistants. She also developed a new Practical Nursing Program at Anoka Technical College and was its Director, before becoming Vice-President of the College for over twenty years. She also taught teaching skills to Vocational teachers for many years. She has written extensively, including ten editions of *Textbook of Basic Nursing.*

Caroline was originator of the Float Pool at Minneapolis General Hospital and has done rescue and general staff nursing, as well as School Nursing. She was Executive Director of the Minnesota Lions' Eye Bank and Director of the Public Health Nursing Department in Wright County, Minnesota. After retiring from Anoka, she was a nurse in Inpatient Psychiatry at Hennepin County Medical Center for over twenty years.

Caroline has a very busy life. She is married to Ron Christensen. Together, they had four children, one of whom is deceased. They have nine grandchildren and several great-grandchildren. (Three of the grandchildren are pursuing health-related careers.)

Caroline has been active in bands since fourth grade and was the oldest person to march in the University of Minnesota Band. She plays for tailgaters at home football games and is in a summer band. She is also in a Community Band and marches with her grandchildren for Minnesota Homecoming.

She belongs to a number of organizations, including American MENSA, Delta Kappa Gamma Society for Women in Education, and the Psychiatry Advisory Committee at the U of Minnesota. She loves to knit and organized a Prayer Shawl group for her church.

Caroline and Ron own antique cars and participate in many parades. They have won many awards, including several National Gold awards.

She played softball for many years and even umpired an official High School game when the umpire didn't come. She coached her son's Baseball and Football teams (the only woman coach) and was on a trap shooting team. She bowls, plays golf, and enjoyed snowmobiling, skiing, canoeing, backpacking, and competitive sailing.

Caroline has rescued a number of orphaned animals and also won many ribbons and trophies with her champion Black Labradors. She even had a pet skunk named Petunia (who was in several parades.)

She has traveled to all fifty US states and Puerto Rico and has visited over forty-five countries.

This current book contains stories of Caroline's very diverse life as a nurse. Some stories are sad, but many are humorous. We hope you enjoy this book and realize the myriad of opportunities open to the nurse. Thank you to Caroline for her service.